wishing you
love, health, prosperity
and — the most precious gift
of all — time to enjoy them.

to

from

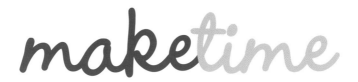

maketime

*A survival guide for women
with too much to do*

Pamela Allardice

A Sue Hines Book
Allen & Unwin

A Sue Hines Book
Allen & Unwin Pty Ltd
83 Alexander Street
Crows Nest NSW 2065
Australia
Phone: (61 2) 8425 0100
Fax: (61 2) 9906 2218
Email: info@allenandunwin.com
Web: www.allenandunwin.com

National Library of Australia
Cataloguing-in-publication entry:
Allardice, Pamela, 1958–.
     Make time.
     ISBN 1 74114 150 8.
     1. Self-care, Health. 2. Time management. I. Title.
     613

Cover & text design by MAU Design
Typesetting by Pauline Haas
Printed in Australia by BPA Printgroup
10 9 8 7 6 5 4 3 2 1

The publisher thanks Corporate Culture
(www.corporateculture.com.au) for the
generous loan of the Fritz Hansen Egg Chair,
designed by Arne Jacobsen.

To my mother – a very busy woman – who has become an excellent gardener, competent nurse, imaginative cook, splendid seamstress, inspired embroiderer, reliable source of all sorts of general information, adequate accountant, fine flower arranger, clever decorator, native wildlife enthusiast, blisteringly rapid stenographer, amateur photographer, and tireless bargain hunter. She has always believed it is possible to get everything done and still have time for herself.

Life is what we make it;
always has been, always will be.

GRANDMA MOSES (NEE ANNA MARY ROBERTSON), PRIMITIVE ARTIST

Contents

Introduction

You need not feel guilty about not being able to keep your life perfectly balanced. Juggling everything is too difficult. All you really need to do is catch it before it hits the floor.

CAROL BARTZ, PRESIDENT AND CEO OF AUTODESK INC.

'There aren't enough hours in the day!' Does this sound familiar? If so, you're probably one of the millions of women – who are also wives, mothers, cooks, financial planners, housekeepers, friends, lovers, caregivers, decision makers and workers – who are struggling to find time for everything. And, unlike men who mostly only have to face time management problems at work, you probably do it around the clock!

I've combined raising two lemme-at-him gimme-my-switchblade types of boys with running a household and sometimes working 50-hour weeks in my business, so I'm familiar with how it feels to grapple with an over-committed life. There have been many days when I've hurled myself out of bed at 6 am and just run flat out all day, without a break, finally collapsing over the finish line at 11 pm. If this sounds like you, it's time to get a grip and get organised. The ability to get more done in less time isn't slavery to work, it's *freedom*. Life is easier, more pleasant and less frustrating when you're organised. You're still going to have the same big pile of stuff to do every day, whether you want to or not, but if you're organised, you can get it done and have plenty of time left over for yourself.

This book is about making the juggling act that is a 21st century woman's life, work. It's about practical action steps and simple, timesaving strategies that will straighten up all areas of your life and put you in charge. And it's not just about making lists and setting goals. Those tools are invaluable, but if you take one thing away from reading this book, I hope it is that the single most critical factor in managing your time is to decide what is vital and important to you. Then you can enjoy and cope better with the essential stuff of life, big and small, good and not-so-good. Sometimes all we can do is share stories about what's really going on in our lives, whether it's caring for an elderly parent, dealing with anxiety or just bracing yourself for a family get-together. Knowing that other women go through what you're going through – and come out stronger and more capable – can give you hope.

I hope that *Make Time* helps you simplify your life and cut back on the non-essential activities that leave you stressed; decrease the relentless 'hurry-up' nature of your life; and make you feel well-prepared for anything life tosses your way. You'll know you've succeeded in combining all the work, home, fun and personal aspects of your life into a satisfying whole when you're enjoying every precious minute.

What do women want? Not much, really. Women want men, careers, money, children, friends, luxury, comfort, independence, freedom, respect, love, and a three-dollar pantyhose that won't run.

PHYLLIS DILLER, COMEDIENNE AND ACTRESS

Advantage: female

Live smarter, not harder

Life is not a dress rehearsal. This is it.

TRADITIONAL

If you're always running out of time, or think you haven't got enough time, it's an interesting exercise to take a step back and think about what time really is. Time is a non-renewable resource, it is irreplaceable, something that will never come again. Therefore, we can't actually 'save' it, 'manage' it or 'make more' of it – we can only spend it. We can, however, manage *ourselves*. In fact, when we fail to do so, that is when events control us and we 'run out of time'. Try these tips:

Try not to distort problems View the curve balls in life as challenges and opportunities rather than as threats to be feared.

Set priorities There is a very fine line between failing and succeeding. People who fail often work just as hard as those who succeed. The major difference is that successful people are more productive. The failures spin their wheels and don't focus.

Assess your choices Too often, all we see are problems. You feel pushed and pulled by fate, helpless. It doesn't have to be this way: there are always things you can do that will make a significant difference to your understanding or attitude, and, therefore, to your actions. The traffic's foul? Leave home 15 minutes earlier and have breakfast in town. Your kids are letting you down? Time for a talk.

Be effective, not just efficient It's possible to be efficient – to process lots of tasks, for example – yet not be effective. An effective person achieves the right results at home or at work with minimum fuss. They are clear about their overriding purpose and daily objectives, and don't waste time on activities that don't support that purpose. There's no point in being efficient if you're efficiently doing the wrong things! The foundation of good time management is finding out what matters deeply to you – what it is you really want to achieve in life.

Feel in control Set realistic goals and, if necessary, readjust those goals to make them attainable.

 START RESPONDING IN A SLIGHTLY DIFFERENT WAY to any set of circumstances and you can alter their effects.

Take a soul break

Don't put off the things you really want to do because life has a way of, well, getting in the way. What do you really want to do? Everything? Nothing? I think that what most women yearn for, more than anything, is time. Time to think. Time to play. Time to waste. Instead of aiming for a trip or a treat, give yourself time off. A day, a month, even a weekend. It's less about the length of time you have away, and more about how you use it. You shouldn't assume the hardest part will be the logistics of making room in your schedule. It's far more likely to be emotional roadblocks that trip you up: other people's expectations, even criticism, and your own guilt. Figuring out a way to take a break is often easier than you think. Here's how:

Focus on the positive Instead of thinking of all the reasons why you can't take a break, direct your energies towards thinking about what you'd like to do. Go to Wales? Trek around New Zealand? Whatever it is, read books, do Internet research. Fear of taking a risk is often the greatest impediment to getting what you want.

Talk to other people who've done it Don't just ask about how wonderful the camping trip to Uluru or cooking class in Provence was. Pose nitty-gritty questions: 'Who paid your bills while you were away?' 'What did you do with your dog?'

No money? Look into grants, fellowships, scholarships, tax-deductible conferences, and house-swapping. There's always a way.

Be informed Find out your company's policy (official or unofficial) on leave and sabbaticals. Be prepared to explain how the company will benefit – or at least, not suffer – from what you propose to do.

Get everyone on board Loved ones and co-workers may feel envious or upset by the potential disruption to their lives. Try to involve family members in the planning process; stress how much happier you – and therefore they – will feel if you explore your dream.

It doesn't have to be long A week-long or even a weekend retreat to a spa or beach-side cottage can be as revitalising as a longer break – and a lot easier to manage.

 DO SOMETHING SPECIAL. If a break is out of the question, at least make a full year's commitment to a life-affirming activity or skill that won't disrupt your routine. Running off to France might not be on the cards – but you could sign up for French lessons.

Look after yourself

Picture this: a man is working in an office; his boss asks him to stop what he's doing and run an Internet search for information to go into the boss's boardroom presentation, pronto. The man does this, knowing it will mean staying back and/or taking his other work home to finish. As the boss goes into the boardroom, he also asks the man to pick up his dry-cleaning, take his messages, and do another Internet search for some backup data. What is wrong with this picture? Well, it is far more likely for a woman to go above and beyond the call of duty when it comes to helping people. They're also far more likely to agree to co-workers' requests to take messages, clear away cups and run errands, irrespective of their position. On the one hand, it may be part of your job to assist in all sorts of extra-curricular activities, and it's also part of being a caring human being to want to help people out on occasion. The critical thing is not to feel that you *always* have to be the one to put up your hand and do jobs that other people can't or won't do.

✳ KNOW THE DIFFERENCE between when you're asked to help out in special circumstances and when you're being taken advantage of.

Say 'no'

I have yet to hear a man ask for advice on how to combine a marriage and a career.

GLORIA STEINEM, AUTHOR AND FOUNDER OF *MS*

Not wanting to let anyone down, not wanting to be seen as stupid or incapable of doing something, and wanting to please (or, at least, not to upset) others are three reasons why women will still say 'yes' when they really shouldn't be taking on any extra responsibilities. I've certainly fallen prey to a heightened sense of responsibility. I've also met and worked with people who quite deliberately set out to find these trigger points in others so they can manipulate them – that's how effective these points are! Practise saying: 'Is this the best use of my time right now?' You may still feel torn, but you are less vulnerable to emotional blackmail when you remind yourself of your real priorities. These tips will also help:

Slowly count to ten Don't answer straightaway if you're put on the spot for an immediate yes or no answer.

Look past the emotional aspects Overlook any feelings of obligation, for example, or even the potential for experiencing satisfaction or achievement, and assess it in terms of cost to your time. Before saying 'yes' or 'no', add up how many hours or days are involved.

Briefly explain your reasons Even if they walk off in a huff, they'll remember why you refused.

Believe, deep down, in your right to say 'no' Conquer the habit of saying 'yes' to every request or obligation when your energy is at stake. Remind yourself that your health comes first, and that taking on too much can compromise your immune system.

 OFFER ALTERNATIVES. Depending on who's asking the favour, and how keen you are to keep the lines of communication open, offer a sweetener: 'No, I can't help out with the invitations – but I'm happy to do the seating plan next week.'

It's not easier to do it yourself

I base everything on the idea that all men are basically just seven years old.

JOAN COLLINS, ACTRESS

Whether you're a high-powered money market analyst or a mother of four who works part-time in a bra shop, there's one thing you'll probably have in common with many other women – you'll be hopeless at delegating tasks. Women are notorious for wanting to handle every detail of a project themselves. If you're serious about getting things done more efficiently, you must learn to trust other people's abilities to do a job. These suggestions will help you delegate more effectively:

Divide a piece of paper into three columns In the first column, list the jobs at work and at home that you could possibly delegate in any given week. Repetitive, routine tasks are the most critical ones. In the second column, mark next to each job the name of a person or organisation to which you could possibly delegate a task. In the third column, write a time when you could brief them about the job – and stick to it.

Explain requests Spell out what you want them to do and how you want it to be done, clearly and concisely. Take into account their abilities (e.g. age, other commitments, speed at which they work) and match your expectations accordingly.

Ask for solutions, not explanations If someone begins to give you a lengthy explanation as to why a task can't be done, resist the urge to say, 'Give it to me and I'll fix it'. Say instead, 'I trust you to look after the details. Just fix the problem'. Or ask, 'If I wasn't here, what would you do?' Chances are, they'll figure it out on their own.

Be patient Don't be overly critical. Your aim is to guide the person and teach them how to do something for you so that you don't have to do it – not to nit-pick or show them how incompetent they are compared to you.

Get out of the way! You can be around to check that a task did get done, and to show appreciation. But if you hover nearby it's a strong signal that you don't trust them to get it right. They will lose interest because they don't feel responsible for the work, and guess who will end up with the ball firmly back in their court?

 DELEGATE TASKS. Other people may not do a job *exactly* or as *perfectly as* the way that you would, but you'll wind up with pretty much the same result.

Marry yourself before you marry anyone else. Promise first to love you, honour you, take care of you and never abandon you.

SARK, POET AND ARTIST

Nurture selectively

Being a mother is like the modern stonewashing process for denim jeans. You may start out crisp, neat and tough, but you end up pale, limp and wrinkled.

KERRY CUE, COMEDIENNE

One of my earliest memories is of when I was about seven years old. There was a boy in our class who was having difficulty with his spelling and, as I was a good speller, the teacher made him sit next to me so that I could help him. Now, on the face of it, it was a great arrangement – he did better, I felt proud of myself and my work didn't suffer. However, interestingly, there was another boy in the class who was an excellent speller, probably better than me, but no one asked him to take care of other students. Why? Because, as my teacher told me, 'Girls are better at helping others than boys are'.

Whether you subscribe to the view that nurturing is something that is inherent to the female, or whether it's something that is learned and encouraged, there's nothing at all wrong with wanting to take care of someone or something because you love them and want to help out. As a woman, being people-oriented is a great strength and one that works to your advantage in managing your time, because you are sensitive to your environment. However, it can get out of control if you get distracted and give-give-give constantly, until you've run dry.

 PUT A TIME LIMIT ON THE NEXT FAVOUR YOU DO for someone of, say, 30 minutes, and stop when you reach the allotted time.

Take a healthy dose of scepticism

Not so long ago I poured the first of my two much-loved daily cups of coffee and opened the newspaper to the headline, 'New study finds coffee unlikely to cause heart problems'. Just for a lark I went and looked up a clipping from a month or so prior that said, 'Study shows heart risk leaps with four cups of coffee daily'. Newspapers do this all the time. When it comes to the latest scientific findings on lifestyle, relationships, and diet and nutrition, the articles flip and flop like a fish on the floor of a boat. Here's how to separate the sense from the nonsense:

Count the legs Research done only on four-legged species doesn't mean a lot for humans. Pregnant rats, for instance, are more likely than humans to bear offspring with missing toes after getting extremely high jolts of caffeine.

Ask how many guinea pigs there were The best research uses at least 100 subjects, preferably more, in order to be statistically significant. Therefore, you should look askance at a study showing that eating 19 tiny meals a day lowers cholesterol and helps you lose weight, if there were only 11 participants.

Find out who's paying for it There's a big difference between papers delivered at company-funded conferences and papers published in medical journals. After all, if the bills are being paid by a big pharmaceutical company, why should you be surprised to find that the researchers have found something good to say about the product?

Wait for confirmation Don't let one study change your life. I look for three things when it comes to food research. First, I check large studies that show a link between a food item and good or bad health – Italy's big appetite for olive oil, and its low rate of heart disease, for instance. I then look for lab evidence that suggests how that food might cause its effect in people. Finally, I check for human studies in which two groups are compared, one eating the food, the other not.

 DON'T SACRIFICE PLEASURE. I apply this rule to my own meals. I skimp on butter and favour olive oil; I eat plenty of fruit and vegetables, lots of potatoes, rice, beans, and pasta, and modest amounts of lean meat; and I have a 375 g pack of freshly ground espresso coffee, or what's left of it, in the fridge. Good health is one of life's great treasures – but so is good food.

Settle for 85 per cent

Men tend to take the 'big picture' approach, cutting straight to the chase and looking to end results such as summaries, charts, final costs and plans. A woman tends to pore over every detail leading up to the end result. This is why we're also prone to feeling panicked and overwhelmed, and to thinking that we'll never get the task finished, let alone started.

Perfectionism is a recipe for anxiety, depression and stress. People who feel they're always failing can't help but be nervous wrecks. Realise that if you spread your energies too thin and your performance suffers, you won't even come close to your own high standards. Instead, tell yourself you'll be happy if you achieve a next-to-perfect 'score'. To get 85 per cent of most projects and activities right is usually good enough. That doesn't mean you deliberately make errors or give less than your best. It does mean you stop polishing and fiddling, and that you don't agonise over the fact you're not spending more time on it. Create it, check it, then let it go.

BE EXCELLENT, NOT PERFECT. Even in the most disappointing situation, try to look for some small way in which you did succeed: 'The food was awful, but everyone had a great time anyway.'

Be proactive

I run my company according to feminine principles – principles of caring; making intuitive decisions; not getting hung up on hierarchy or all those dreadfully boring business-school management ideas; having a sense of work as being part of your life, not separate from it; putting your labour where your love is; being responsible to the world in how you use your profits; recognising the bottom line should stay at the bottom.

ANITA RODDICK, FOUNDER OF THE BODY SHOP

People who take control of their circumstances, who attend to the important activities instead of allowing urgent, but unimportant, items to run their lives, are proactive. They are less likely to feel out of control, pushed and pulled by the winds of fate. Also, if the current way of doing things is not working for them, they will actively look for improved methods, rather than just accepting the existing protocol as the best and only way. Proactive behaviour is anything that will make a significant long-term difference in your life: weekly and daily planning, long-term planning, preventing crises, studying, cultivating new directions and interests, developing relationships, enjoying recreation.

A reactive person, on the other hand, passively accepts what comes their way, even when they don't like it. Most of us spend at least half of our day in 'reactive' mode, dealing with phone calls and unexpected visitors, not to mention any sort of crisis, deadline, or putting out of fires because something wasn't done properly the first time around. Reactive people are less likely to reach beyond what is immediately clamouring for their attention in order that they can tackle other issues that will actually make a bigger difference.

MASTER BEING PROACTIVE, and you master yourself.

Ask for help

Our greatest glory is not in never failing, but in being humble enough to ask for help when we fail.

CONFUCIUS, CHINESE PHILOSOPHER

Why do so many otherwise sane women have this pathological aversion to appearing to be needy? Feeling overwhelmed makes it more imperative than ever that we ask for help. Here are some of the most common reasons why we don't, and how to counteract them:

Independence is not the same as fending for yourself The women in my family are from pioneer stock – capable, warm-hearted and red-headed (some would say, uncharitably, hard-headed). 'Do it yourself', was their catch-cry. However, being able to take care of yourself and your family properly means accepting that sometimes you do need help. Employing a cleaner doesn't make you a damsel in distress.

You don't want to be weak Perhaps you want to be seen as a reliable, responsible person. Yet trying to do it all actually undermines your effectiveness. It's far better to be realistic about what you can accomplish. Set limits and delegate early and often.

You hate owing anyone anything If you feel you will be obligated to someone if they do something for you, you're seeing the situation as a way a person can assert power over you – and you're probably selling your relationships short. Start by asking for help from those for whom you can do simple favours back.

You don't deserve help Ooh, I smell burning martyr! It's time to put on that tiara and develop a sense of entitlement, whether that means hiring a painter or getting the groceries delivered instead of hauling them yourself – just because you can do something doesn't mean you have to.

You are asking, but no one is listening Are you asking clearly enough? If you're feeling defensive while making a request, it can come across camouflaged with all sorts of 'I don't really need you', 'Don't worry about it', signals.

WORK OUT WHAT YOU'RE WORTH. If you earn an annual salary, calculate your hourly wage. Then, perhaps you can pay someone else less than your rate to do some of the chores you hate the most.

If they don't know, they can't do it

'I hate having to wait until the rubbish needs to be taken out and then asking my husband to take it out', says one friend. 'Why can't he do it *before* I ask?' Many women secretly believe that if people around them truly cared, they'd notice when help was needed. In fact, a good relationship isn't about reading someone else's mind, it's about being able to share your thoughts – so ask. Here are some tips to help you let everyone know what's expected of them so you don't have to keep nagging:

List all the jobs that need to be done regularly For example, meal planning, shopping, cooking, housework, folding laundry, putting out garbage, childcare, gardening, watering plants, family-related paperwork and bill-paying, repairs, helping with homework, after-school activities, car maintenance, feeding pets, and household errands. Have sub-headings under each job. For example, for housework write vacuuming, dusting, making beds, and tidying up.

Next to each sub-heading, write who does most of it Is it you, or someone else? If your name appears the most often, then this is a pretty clear indication that the division of work in your household isn't fair.

Make new house rules Agree on which tasks each of you think are important. Then, taking into account the abilities of everyone in the household, redraw the list to reflect a more equal allocation of tasks. Make it clear that each of you will pick up the others' responsibilities during times of crisis – but only then.

Put up a chart Write each person's name on it and the chores they have to do, then put it where it can't be missed – the fridge is a time-honoured spot, but a wipe-clean bulletin board in the kitchen is a longer-lasting option.

Resist criticism Accept that other people may not do tasks as thoroughly as you do. If you criticise people, they'll be less likely to help in the future – and don't go over the job and do it again!

 TRAIN UP YOUR SUBORDINATES. If you avoid delegating jobs to your family because it takes too long and they don't do things properly, make the time to show them exactly how you want things done. The pay-off is that kids learn a skill, get a sense of responsibility, and feel as though they are a valued member of your family team.

Stop catastrophising

You can't worry about what might happen to you tomorrow. You get spastic enough worrying about what's happening right now.

LAUREN BACALL, ACTRESS

Society expects us to be in control no matter what is thrown at us in an average day: keeping a $250 000 client happy, making a speech to 100 heard-it-all-before sales reps with a wonky microphone, or catching a plane. A certain amount of fretting and cautiousness is essential for the survival of the species. But breaking out in a sweat at the thought of driving to the city, or anguishing over what might or might not befall your child, doesn't do anyone any good. The following behavioural habits all feed anxiety:

Jumping to conclusions Women tend to have a low opinion of themselves, so they often think others do too. Instead of assuming the worst, get a reality check. When seeking feedback, avoid assigning blame. Instead of, 'You think I'm unambitious and antisocial', try, 'I think you're annoyed because I wanted to leave early. Is that so?'

Seeing the world in black and white All-or-nothing thinking leaves little room for error, should you, or others, very naturally fall short. Watch for words such as 'never', 'must', 'should' and 'always'.

Taking things personally Anxious people often believe they are responsible for everyone else's happiness and comfort. By association they assume that everyone else's misery is their fault too. Challenge such thoughts.

 FACE YOUR DEMONS. 'Free-floating anxiety' – that which doesn't appear to have any noticeable cause – may be due to a personal secret. It takes an awful lot of mental energy to make sure that you keep a secret and that no one guesses it. If this rings true, seek out a therapist or support group, and offload the burden.

Take a punt in life, that's what I believe.
If you just sit there the days run away.
If you make a few mistakes, who cares?
You can shut yourself in your house
and never come out again, or you
can hang in there and keep on trying.
You decide which.

LADY RUPERT CLARKE

Know your strengths

Working mothers often feel as though they are walking a tightrope between the cultures of the housewife and the working man.

ARLIE HOCHSCHILD, AUTHOR

Several typically female traits can support your quest to find time and to organise your life better. Acknowledge their presence within you, and practise using them more often:

Use your woman's intuition This phrase is often bandied about, but rarely in connection with its ability to solve problems. Paying special attention to what that little inner voice is telling you and really hearing and empathising with what others have to say, can help you make the right decisions. Men, by comparison, tend to look for an answer straightaway, analyse facts and figures, and come straight to a 'logical' conclusion.

Mull it over Women tend to take suggestions on board and think them over until they 'feel right', which can result in reaching more holistic, consensual outcomes at work and at home. A woman's ability to talk about problems and issues, and to get others to open up and share ideas, can contribute not only to a more pleasant home life, but to fewer work-related misunderstandings.

Use the power of flexibility Women can and do handle more than one person or situation simultaneously. We also tend to be more adaptable and go with the flow, while men tend to lock their focus on a job and not stop until they've finished.

 DAYDREAM. It is not a waste of time – quite the opposite. Let yourself daydream while you walk the dog, hang out washing or drive. When your mind wanders, you often find new ideas and solutions to problems.

… and your greatest weakness

*I am haunted wherever I go, day or night, by the idea that
every other mother is calmer and less selfish than I.*

ADRIENNE RICH, POET

Most working mothers still suffer a tremendous burden of guilt at not living up to
the 1950s picket-fence-and-frilly-apron myth of what a mother should be like. In the
1946 edition of *Dr Spock's Baby and Child Care*, the best-selling bible on childcare at
the time, Spock warned that, 'It doesn't make much sense to have mothers go to work
and have them pay other people to do a poorer job of bringing up their children'.
Even when, 40 years later he grudgingly conceded, 'Both parents have an equal right
to a career if they want one, and an equal obligation to share in the care of their
children', no one told parents how to accomplish it.

The dilemmas of modern motherhood arise from a mismatch between the current
realities of family life and ideas about mothers and children that stem from the late
19th and early 20th centuries. Women feel guilty that they cannot be with their
children more, that their housekeeping is slipshod and that their substitute childcare
may not be good enough. They even feel guilty when their children's behaviour
shows the ups and downs of normal development. And should anything truly go
awry for their children, others are only too eager to wag their fingers at the working
mother – particularly if she's a single parent! Why does little Johnny get into trouble
for fighting at school? Because his mum works, of course. What about all the children
who are having problems whose mothers are at home? And what about Johnny's
father?

Accept that it is simply impossible to be Superwoman. In fact, in many ways,
today's Superwoman is Everywoman. The only way to 'have it all' is not to try to do it
all. When a son needs a cuddle or a daughter needs help with her school project, the
kitchen floor may not get swept. But every gritty footstep will be a reminder of the
things that really matter.

 DON'T BEAT YOURSELF UP about things you can't change – learn lessons for the
future instead.

Tune into your rhythms

Man can work till set of sun – but woman's work is never done.

TRADITIONAL

Everyone has certain times in the day when they're more alert and so perform better. Think about your pattern of physical and mental energy levels, then try to adjust your daily schedule to mesh with it. By handling mentally demanding jobs during your peak energy periods, you can get more done in less time. Are you a morning person or a night owl? If you're a night owl, burning the midnight oil may result in maximum productivity for you. If you're an early bird, get up early and start working while everyone else in your house is still asleep. If you don't feel that you're either, choose the morning. When you start early you can complete a significant amount of your day's work quota by the time others are first stumbling into their offices. You can then finish the day's work early and have the rest of the time to either do more work or to play. Late starters are behind from the minute they get up, and feel increasing pressure to get their work done as the hour grows even later.

TRY 'DAWNLIGHTING'. You've heard of 'moonlighting', or working a second job in the evening. Well, if there's something that needs doing, whether it's walking the dog or checking a report, consider the peace and quiet of early morning before everyone else gets up.

Coping as you care

They say that you have to have a personal stake in a subject to be able to speak about it. Certainly, until about a year ago, I would have felt somewhat immune to the difficulties of caring for a friend or family member, especially an elderly relative. Then my aunt had a partial stroke and went into a nursing home: the same intrepid, spirited woman who had been school dux, artist's model, philanthropist and world traveller. Nothing could have prepared me for how devastating it is to see a loved one become less than they once were. Showing that you care is important, as is devoting time to your loved one. But so it doesn't take a toll on you, rendering you useless to all (including yourself), here are few things my experience has taught me:

Determine treatment options If it's clear that a loved one is seriously ill, discuss with them what they do and do not want with regard to their care while you still can. If they don't want to talk about it, or can't understand, share the responsibility with friends and relatives.

Insist on helping Even if the loved one – or the main caregiver, if it's not you – refuses, you should still insist. They won't be able to manage alone.

Stay in touch Designate one family member to relay updates to others. Call the main caregiver frequently and give them a chance to blow off steam. Take turns relieving them – even a week's break from visiting can be an enormous relief.

Establish a relationship with the doctor Be very precise when talking to doctors. They don't necessarily volunteer information, so make a list of questions in order of importance. It may be that there are questions you don't want to ask in front of the patient, in which case you'll need to make an appointment for a phone or face-to-face consultation. Get to know the nurses and social workers. Often they are more comfortable dealing with the emotional side of situations.

Listen to what your loved one says If it is your mum or dad, you may feel as though you have become the parent, but you haven't. As long as they are mentally competent, they have the right to make their own decisions, even if you don't approve.

 ASK FOR HELP. When you feel overwhelmed, enlist help. Don't be afraid to ask – it's one of the things family and friends are there for.

Anticipate crises

I am first and last a wife and mother, which means that I can lose up to half of any given day when one son has invited the baseball team over after training, the other son has a project due tomorrow, and when Doug has invited his friend who is in town for the evening to come for dinner. Working women – especially working mothers – must have contingency plans. It's vital to be able to think ahead and ask yourself: 'What if such-and-such happened?' If you get into the habit of anticipating what to do in unexpected situations, you will always rise to the occasion with a plan when (not if!) the crisis happens. For example:

Have backup childcare Make up a list of reliable babysitters and helpful family members or neighbours. If you have a partner, it's only fair that you work out a white-knuckled agreement for when things get derailed thanks to a chickenpox outbreak at school. Perhaps he stays home with a sick child in the morning while you go to work, then you relieve him at lunchtime. Obviously a lot depends on your work, but splitting your time is a saner option than the responsibility falling on you.

Keep an emergency meal in the freezer That way, anyone taking over for you can just heat it up quickly. A hearty soup or casserole plus garlic bread makes a good nourishing dinner. Have extra non-perishables on hand in case of emergencies, e.g. baked beans, tomato sauce, sugar. You'll always use them, so they won't go to waste.

Draw up a master list of household information For example, when rubbish collection days fall and where spare keys are, just in case someone has to step in for you. This list should also include important phone numbers of family and friends, plus kids' mobile numbers, after-school care, babysitter, doctor, poisons information service, dentist, vet, school, electrician, gardener, hospital, plumber, taxi, police, fire brigade, chemist, ambulance, next-door neighbour, etc. Tape it to the inside of your pantry door or keep it in a protective plastic sleeve on the kitchen noticeboard so everyone in the house knows about it. Put a pad and pen next to the telephone for taking messages.

Keep emergency money Hide a small amount of cash in a secure place to give your family enough money to tide them over should you be called away.

 KEEP A SENSE OF PERSPECTIVE. Today's crisis is tomorrow's history. So do the best you can, and try not to worry, as it never solves anything.

Schedule 'me' time

Put it in your diary, as if it were a doctor's appointment. Whether it's shopping, going for a facial or simply relaxing guilt-free with a magazine, make quality time for yourself. Most of us are better time managers than we realise. But often we don't create time just to veg out, as we're too busy being busy. However, time-out is vital as it allows you to recharge your batteries. Try these ideas:

Fit in time-outs To avoid tension buildup, follow this rule: for every 50 minutes you work, take a 5-minute break. Time-outs are proven to increase productivity.

Take your holidays Austrian researchers have proven that even a one-week holiday does more than just clear the mind and calm the spirit – it also improves health and reduces stress levels for up to five weeks. Both during and after a good holiday, we sleep better and enjoy better moods.

Meditate It offers a gentle way to slow you down during a hectic day. Even if you can't see yourself sitting cross-legged and saying 'om', you can still learn to achieve focus and relaxation – the real essence of meditating. Sit comfortably in a place where you will not be disturbed. Close your eyes, or keep them open and softly focussed on something in front of you. Pay attention to your breathing. Notice how your stomach expands and contracts as you inhale and exhale. If troubling thoughts enter your mind, simply return your focus to your breathing. Practise this exercise for about 15 minutes every day.

 PLAN A WEEKEND OF COMPLETE R'N'R. Look ahead in your calendar and find a weekend that is uncommitted and schedule some Rest and Relaxation. Draw a line through it and plan to wake up on the Saturday morning and do whatever you feel like doing for fun (no chores allowed!).

Planning essentials
The bag

Women are much more torn than men – in any given 24 hours – to meet all their commitments and achieve their objectives for that day. Want proof? Just watch men and women on the street or in shopping centres. Most men will be carrying either nothing, or one simple briefcase. Women, on the other hand, will be carrying a handbag, as well as a briefcase, possibly a couple of shopping bags, even a baby bag. Why? It's because women not only do so many jobs for people they look after or work with, they also need to be able to connect to anyone or anything at any time.

Make your carry-everywhere bag work for you, so that you've got all the information and supplies you need, wherever you go. Bags with several zippered compartments work best. If you use a mobile phone, get a bag that has a special outside pocket for it to slide into. Clean out your bag regularly and get rid of things that don't belong in there. Keep receipts for business expenses in one section of your handbag or wallet, and file them daily. Here's a checklist for your handbag basics:

A diary, appointment calendar, Filofax or electronic organiser Choose one with a roomy section for each day and a section for addresses and phone numbers. Write all appointments in your diary, not on bits of paper.

A mobile phone, a to-do list for that day, at least two pens, a small calculator, and a small notepad or tear-off Post-it notes

Wallet or billfold Make sure it has sections for cash, licence, business cards, credit and health insurance cards. Make a list of all the items in your wallet including credit card numbers and keep it in a separate place. This will make it easier to replace everything quickly, should your bag be lost or stolen. Buy a brightly coloured wallet, such as red, so you can see it immediately, even if you haven't got your glasses on.

A personal survival kit Buy miniature sizes of lip balm, hand cream, mirror or powder compact, tissues, tampons, safety pins and bandaids.

Car and home keys Put them in the same spot every time you put them in your bag, preferably in an outside zippered pocket, so you can reach them with one hand. Buy a fluorescent key ring so you can see keys immediately, even when it's dark.

The phone

The telephone is probably the single most powerful tool at your disposal for getting your home and work life better organised, yet it is often the most misused. Here are some ideas for using your phone more efficiently and effectively:

Shop for sensible features Buy a phone with push-button dialling otherwise you probably won't be able to negotiate many companies' voicemail systems.

Caller ID This display feature that identifies the source of incoming calls means you can decide whether to take a call, or let voicemail handle it.

Memory dial It is an option that allows you to store frequently-dialled numbers and activate them with the push of one button.

Voicemail Choose voicemail rather than an answering machine because it continues to work even if there's a power failure. Look for a plan that lets you retrieve messages from phones other than your own.

Call waiting A tone lets you know that someone else is dialling and, by pressing a key, you can put the first call on hold and check who is on the line.

Good manners and commonsense go a long way Answer your calls promptly – you sound (and feel) more responsive and alert if you do so. Identify yourself – give your name and telephone number. Train your kids to do the same. When you are making a call, be upfront and give as much information about yourself as possible: 'Hello, it's Pamela Allardice for James Big-shot, I'm calling about donating a prize for the school trivia night.' This way you avoid offensive and time-wasting screening questions from the other person.

Take messages It sounds simple, but so few people can do it properly! Taking accurate messages avoids confusion and ensures that calls can be returned promptly. Listen carefully to the caller, and write down everything important – their name, the time they called, their telephone number and the message, if any.

Be nice Everyone has bad days, but try not to take them out on the person who's called you. My father taught me always to answer the phone with a smile on my face – corny as it may be, it does make you sound more pleasant and alert.

Keep it short Brief calls save time. When you are about to make a call, write down the main points you need to cover, checking them off as you discuss them. This will stop you getting sidetracked.

Goals are dreams with deadlines.

DIANA SCHARF HUNT, AUTHOR

Setting goals

Get a new attitude

If you think you can, you're right.
And if you think you can't, you're right.

MARY KAY ASH, FOUNDER OF MARY KAY COSMETICS

Speak to any woman on any subject and pretty soon she'll say something like, 'I always feel as though I'm falling behind, I just can't seem to catch up', or, 'I'm so tired from being on the go all the time; I'm constantly being pulled in too many directions'. As if these self put-downs weren't bad enough, there's a sinister subtext to them too: that is, seeing as you can't even finish all the jobs that should be done, you certainly haven't got time for pleasant but probably non-essential activities.

No matter how hard and fast you go at any to-do list, you won't get everything done if there's too much on the list in the first place. Get into the habit of ranking priorities; don't regard rolling non-essential activities into the next day as a failure. When next putting together a list of things to do, ask yourself which ones you can cross off or leave for another day. Of course you can't keep putting off the boring or difficult ones forever, but there's bound to be something that you can put on hold. A sure-fire way to gain time is to put only the absolutely essential items on your agenda. Your attitude is bound to shift towards the positive because, instead of chastising yourself at the end of each day for failing to achieve your goals and panicking about how much more you now have to do the next day, you'll be able to say, 'At least I got the really important things done – anything else is a bonus'.

 DON'T GET DISCOURAGED BY A LONG TO-DO LIST. Make it shorter. The most effective managers identify only three top priorities each day. Try it. Your self-esteem gets a big boost when you repeatedly cross off all three tasks, day after day.

Honour your values

A person can be successful in fiscal and material terms, but still be weak and lacking in direction. Some of the most discontented and cynical people I've met are those who believe success is measured by money, expensive toys, the right address or how many influential names they can drop into a conversation.

True personal power comes from within, from basing your life on certain fundamental principles. It comes from the heart and the soul. Consider the analogy of a beautiful garden: in order to create it, it's necessary to prepare the soil thoroughly. Taking a short cut to an attractive conclusion in any situation – whether it's to do with work, family or relationships – is rarely successful in the long-term if that preparatory 'spade-work' hasn't been put in as well. As my mother always used to say, 'We get back what we give out'. Peace of mind and effective living only come through connecting with your own truth, and living by sound values. These are the ones I try to live by, and you can probably add more:

Be positive Take a forward-looking, enthusiastic approach to life.

Act with integrity Know the difference between right and wrong.

Be loyal Support family, friends and colleagues.

Have courage Don't run away when something difficult or disagreeable needs to be done; face up to things.

Learn to be patient Appreciate that it's often going to take several attempts to get something right, and that, in some cases, it's a work-in-progress that's going to take a lifetime.

Be truthful There is no such thing as a good lie, or a lie that doesn't matter.

Show respect In everything you do or say, respect yourself, respect others, be willing to consider others' views, and be responsible for your actions.

HAVE A CLEAR PICTURE OF WHAT MATTERS TO YOU. Every day your actions should put flesh on your dreams, and help you make the right decisions about how you use your time.

Communicate better

If you use the telephone a lot in your work, practise your telephone technique. You'd probably be amazed at how many times you say 'ummm' and 'you know' during each sentence. Then there's the sentences you start, but don't finish and, finally, there's your voice itself. How do you sound? Enthusiastic and upbeat or like a wet dishrag? Try these tips:

Always take a deep breath before you speak on the phone When you have air in your lungs your voice has more depth and power.

Ask yourself, what is the purpose of this call? Spend a few moments thinking about what information you want to obtain or wish to convey and prepare yourself for each call before you make it. Make a list of items you want to discuss with the person you're calling and have files or other papers which you need to refer to close by. Take notes of the conversation when you speak and place them in the file for that job. Even if you've got a good memory it can be difficult to remember exactly what was said. In short, treat each call as if it were a face-to-face meeting.

Get savvy about when to call If your work revolves around the telephone – making sales calls, for instance – you should know that there are certain times during the day when you're most likely to find people sitting at their desks and available to speak to you. As a general rule people are usually in their offices between 9 am and 11 am, and 2 pm and 4 pm, so block out those times in your diary or desk planner and use them to make your calls.

Speak slowly and clearly so the person can understand you If you're leaving a message, it's a good idea to spell out your name as well as say it. 'This is Pamela Allardice, A-L-L-A-R-D-I-C-E.' Don't race through your phone number – preferably, say it twice. Using voicemail and answering machines correctly can make you much more productive because you can share information without actually having to speak to the other person. You can also communicate in non-real time – you don't have to stay awake till 1 am to communicate with someone on the other side of the world, for example.

DON'T PLAY TELEPHONE TAG. It is a big time waster. When you leave a phone message, remember the four Ws: Who called, Why you called, What you want the receiver to do, and When you're available for a return call.

State your purpose

An aim in life is the only fortune worth finding.

ROBERT LOUIS STEVENSON, POET

Victor Frankl, the famous Jewish psychiatrist who survived four concentration camps and wrote *Man's Search for Meaning* (1959), discovered that no matter how appalling external conditions are, when people have a vision of something they still want to do, they keep on surviving against impossible odds. By the same token, when you have a statement of purpose, it follows that you'll see what matters most, what matters least, what you need to change, and how to take those first steps. Having a clear sense of purpose gives you the cutting edge that enables you to achieve your chosen goals. Here's how to make your own personal mission statement:

Attitude What's your attitude like? And what would you like it to be? (e.g. I am a conscientious, caring person.)

Values What are the main principles that dictate your behaviour? (e.g. I will always try to put my family first.)

Skills and expertise What do you do? What are you good at? And what do you want to improve upon? (e.g. I am a devoted mother; I am a trained accountant; I will work to improve my listening skills.)

Position How do others see you? How would you like them to see you? (e.g. I am shy and reserved, but people know that I can always be relied upon.)

Ambitions What are you looking forward to? What do you want to do? (e.g. I would eventually like to run my own consultancy.)

Make your mission statement work for you by rewriting it until you have a maximum of two clear, concise sentences. It's much harder to make a short, focussed statement than it is to waffle on for several paragraphs! When you're happy with it, write it in your diary, or post it where you will see and affirm it, daily if possible. At the end of six months or perhaps a year, you may want to change a key word or phrase, which is the natural result of your mind constantly processing new ideas.

 DRAW UP A MISSION STATEMENT. It provides a means for you to clarify your goals as you move through life.

Do what you love

If you wait, all that happens is that you get older.

LARRY MCMURTRY, NOVELIST

'Your life is terrible and terrific, all at once', an old friend said to me recently. The terrible part seemed clear – I work extremely long hours, and when publishing deadlines are coming up, 12-hour days are the norm. But the terrific part was also obvious – apart from being blessed with two fantastic kids and a loving husband, I actually love what I do.

It hasn't always been this way: I've had several appalling jobs. There was the time when I was working for an egotistical and irresponsible psychiatrist who gave his patients marijuana during counselling sessions because he was curious to see what effect it would have on them. And let's not forget the multinational chemical company that dumped toxins in neighbouring bushland – and that fired me when I reported them to the appropriate authorities.

Many people not only put in horrendous hours, they work for unpleasant or even corrupt bosses, and for companies who do nothing to improve our world. They can't wait to get out the door at the end of the day and their physical, mental and spiritual health all suffer. It would be naive of me to tell anyone to simply 'follow your bliss'. It is rarely that easy and, often, it is only when unsatisfying work gets to the point where it is taking a toll on our health that we will make radical changes to our working lives. Sometimes, taking that terrifying leap of faith into The Great Unknown means things will work out for the best. When I left that high-paying job with the chemical company to work in a health food store, study natural therapies and write books, plenty of people thought I was nuts. Changing jobs is hard, but doing what you love is less stressful, healthier, even downright fun.

 START AN ACCOMPLISHMENT JOURNAL. At the end of each day, jot down one thing you feel good about having accomplished at your job and one thing you feel good about having done for yourself or with friends or family. Reading this diary can help you figure out what is making you happy and what isn't. The patterns you discover will help you make better decisions for the future.

Get networking

The word 'networking' has fallen out of favour, because it's come to mean schmoozing, lobbying and jockeying for position and power. It is, in fact, a much underrated skill and one which most women are extremely good at: talking to other people and, ultimately, finding out how you might be able to help each other. Here's how to network efficiently and positively, without being seen as aggressive:

Check out organisations or clubs There may be more than one that attracts you, in which case, decide which is most relevant. What facilities do they offer? What support services? Having joined, get involved – volunteer for a committee, attend meetings or put your hand up to help organise events.

Carry cards Exchanging business cards remains a critical part of doing business. There's no point in attending a function unless you take some to hand out. Don't be apologetic about offering your card – jump right in!

Don't be self-conscious It took me a long time to overcome my dread of walking into a room full of strangers, whether it was a mothers' group morning tea, or a sales meeting. Like most human beings, I was thinking that everyone was looking at me. Wrong. In fact, most people are also thinking about themselves! To feel more comfortable in a meeting or at a function where you don't know a soul, shift your attention to another person, be interested in them and ask them questions about themselves. Then move on to the next person.

Be open to opportunity Sometimes the best networking and contact-making opportunities are found in the least likely places, at the school canteen, for example, or church, or book club meetings.

Follow up Where appropriate, send a brief note or card to someone you've met, reiterating what you discussed, and emphasising that you'd like to catch up and/or do business.

 PRACTISE DESCRIBING YOURSELF. Try this exercise: stand in front of a mirror. Set a timer for 15 seconds. Now, turn to the mirror and introduce yourself, explaining who you are and what you do in the allocated time. Hard, isn't it? Do it again till you've got it down pat. Don't think of it as a sales pitch, or as showing off – just be positive and upbeat about who you are.

How habits help – and hinder

Good habits are as easy to form as bad ones.

TIM McCARVER, SPORTSCASTER

We've all got them – bad habits that make life more difficult than it needs to be. For me, it was dozing for that extra delicious half hour after the alarm went off, only to wake with a jolt, hurling myself out of bed, feeling flustered before I'd even started the day. By making myself get up at the right time and doing some gentle stretching exercises or taking a walk before having a more leisurely shower, I not only increased my productivity tremendously, I also eliminated a major cause of stress in my life. The following advice will help you move through life more smoothly:

Make a list of your bad habits Whatever they are, once you have identified them, put them on the list. Then put it somewhere you will see it every day, such as on your work noticeboard, or on the fridge door.

Keep it simple Don't feel as though you have to come up with a revolutionary idea for every project you're involved with. Putting pressure on yourself to perform can leave you bogged down in unnecessary details. Many successful solutions in daily life are simply commonsense and are reworked to meet a specific need.

Break up your routine Switch back and forth between different tasks. Arrange your schedule so you can turn from one project to another at least once or twice a day. Try to balance must-do tasks with things that are refreshing, and which challenge you. If most of your daily activities are familiar, aim to focus at least 10 per cent of your time on new projects or ideas.

Don't get distracted Worrying about things that haven't happened yet is a waste of time and energy. Get everything signed-off before starting work.

Set goals – even if you don't need to Without a goal and a deadline, the motivation to do any task is removed. Author Stephen King writes 1500 words every day except on his birthday, Christmas and the 4th of July. If you truly want to meet a deadline and be successful, you need to keep going until you can do no more. Try not to make deadlines too tight – always factor in the unexpected.

 DO THE BEST YOU CAN. Don't worry about whether what you are doing is different or better than what others have done before you.

Be nice to people on your way up –
you will meet them on the way down.

JIMMY DURANTE, ACTOR

Speak with confidence

Giving a speech or presentation is right up at the top of the stress stakes, along with moving house, getting a divorce and coping with bereavement. Here's how to make things a little easier:

Practise, practise, practise Rehearse your speech or presentation so thoroughly that you know it word-perfect, or as close as you can. Another trick is to record yourself and play it back so you can identify weak or cringe-worthy spots to work on.

Be prepared for questions If you know that you are going to receive questions from the floor, spend some time thinking about possible contentious issues that may come up and what you would say.

Be clear about your goal What do you want or need to achieve with your speech? Perhaps it's to inform a group of colleagues about sales figures, or maybe it's to entertain a group of women at a sewing group lunch. Focus on this goal, rather than on your stage fright.

Be beautifully introduced Well ahead of time, send the organisation or group a brief biographical note so that they know how to introduce you appropriately.

Make crib cards Rather than have a bundle of large sheets, write key words for each point on palm-sized cards that will remind you what to talk about. Number them and check they're in the right order before you start.

Check the room first Make sure audiovisual equipment works. Test the microphone, clipping it on if it's a head mike, or adjusting the height if it's a standard.

Take a good look at yourself Are your clothes neat and tidy? Make sure your buttons are buttoned, that your skirt isn't tucked into your pantyhose at the back after a last-minute dash to the toilet, and that you haven't got sticky tape or worse attached to your shoes. Check your teeth for lipstick and spinach. Put your shoulders back, take a deep breath, and smile as you greet your audience.

Steady your hands Either hold onto the bench or lectern, or grip the microphone. Don't hold papers, as they will rustle.

Laugh If things go wrong, and they're bound to sometimes, laugh and start again.

 SPEAK SLOWLY. A common fault is to speak much too fast when you're nervous. Stop and take a breath to emphasise a point. If you have a time limit, place your watch in front of you so you can keep track of the time.

Pulverise procrastination

Procrastination is opportunity's assassin.

VICTOR KIAM, ENTREPRENEUR

The most insidious thing about procrastination is that the job gets bigger and harder the longer you keep putting it off. Once started, it usually doesn't take that long after all. Here's how to stop the rot:

Get the facts When faced with a big task, first set out and review all the available information. If necessary, ask for more. Evaluate several possible outcomes – if two outcomes are close contenders, ask yourself which one has the edge, and why? Which one will be most beneficial for you? If, however, there is no new information to be had, then pull the job out, do it now, and finish it! Quite often, with jobs you keep putting off until later, you may be fearful of 'winging it' with only what you know and are capable of doing without further instruction. In this case, the habit of procrastination is masking your fear that the particular skill you can offer just isn't good enough, so it may be more of a confidence issue than a time management one.

Be prepared to take a risk Sometimes, despite the best intentions and thorough planning, a decision may not turn out for the best. It doesn't matter, at least you've moved from point A to point B. If necessary, you can now make another decision and move to point C. Indecision is unsettling and will undermine your confidence until you end up going neither forwards nor backwards.

Break it down If a job is overwhelming, turn it into a series of steps. Promise yourself you'll spend a set period of time on it – say, an hour – each day till it's done. Schedule these times for quiet periods when there will be few interruptions.

Focus on the outcome Imagine how great you'll feel when the job is completed. Give yourself rewards for getting the job done and/or at the close of each stage.

 STAY FLEXIBLE. All your careful planning will be of little use if you can't veer from the schedule you set. You may have to spend time handling crises. Or you may get on a roll with a particular task, in which case it would be a mistake to stop just because you only scheduled an hour for it. Instead, practise effective procrastination. Ask yourself, 'Is putting off my next scheduled task and continuing what I'm doing a smart decision, or is it just a delay tactic?'

Think more effectively

Why is it that we can be stumped by even the simplest question, given that thought impulses travel in our brains at nearly the speed of light? It has nothing to do with being stupid, and everything to do with learning how to think more efficiently. Here's how:

Know what the problem is How often do you go off half-cocked without knowing what it is you actually want and need to do? Make sure you are in the best possible position to take action or to make a decision before you do so.

Look and listen Whether you're deciding if a teenager can go to a dance, or whether to buy shares in a company, the process should be the same – you must have all the facts so you can make an informed decision.

Think outside the square Solving a problem doesn't mean doing what has always been done before; nor does it mean having to come up with a completely new idea. Sometimes the best decisions are a combination of an old idea and something fresh. Look for synergistic combinations. Are there two projects you're working on that can be rolled together? Can you rearrange your schedule so you don't have two trips in the same direction at different times? Give new ways of doing things a chance. Too many good ideas are killed when we make snap judgements.

Get feedback Getting another person's opinion on an issue can help you focus your thinking and produce solutions you hadn't even thought of. If you still feel you're right, you can of course ignore them, but it's more likely that the feedback will help you come up with the right decision.

Sleep on it Putting a problem or a decision aside for a while is sometimes the only thing to do. Other people may not like the delay, but it's better than making the wrong decision and then having to backtrack. Even if you don't miraculously wake up with the answer, at least you can attack the problem feeling refreshed.

Move your mind Do a crossword puzzle. Read a book. Go to the art gallery. According to a report in *Science News*, the very act of learning creates a 'neural efficiency' that makes it easier for you to think.

 LEARN TO LISTEN PROPERLY. Think about all the time you waste by asking people to repeat things, or by doing something and then realising you misunderstood what you were asked to do. Try taking a 'verbal photograph', saying something like, 'I'll just recap what you're saying so far'.

Be punctual

There will always be days when you're running late through no fault of your own – there was a traffic delay, bad weather or a long line at the checkout. However, being constantly late contributes to that pressurised feeling of never being quite on top of things; plus, from a business point of view, being late sends very negative messages to employers and clients. These tips will get your timing on track:

Keep your word You will feel better about yourself, and certainly feel less stressed. If you say you are going to be somewhere at a certain time, make sure it happens. Even better, be early. Always add ten minutes to however long you think it will take to get somewhere.

Use an alarm clock It sounds obvious, but many people don't – or won't! If you hate being awakened by a loud noise, investigate more attractive-sounding options, such as setting the clock to a classical music station or a tape of nature sounds. Set your alarm for 5 minutes earlier than you really need to.

Wake up happy Train yourself to stretch and say something like, 'This will be a good day', or, 'Whatever happens, I'm going to do my best', before you even stand up. If you don't believe me, try saying something like, 'Damn, raining again, how depressing', before getting up – and see how that affects your day.

Don't sabotage yourself If you know you've got something unpleasant to deal with the next day – perhaps a dentist's appointment or a meeting you'd rather avoid – it's easy simply to do things more slowly because, deep down, you're in no rush! Take a few minutes the night before to face up to what you've got to do in the morning, and say something like, 'I'll get there on time, it'll only take half an hour, and then it's over'. That way, you'll wake up with this affirmation foremost in your mind, and it'll carry you through.

 PLAN AHEAD. Put out the right clothes, make lunches and pack bags the night before, without fail. If you know you're going out after work, factor in 10 minutes before bed to run through your usual evening check-list – if you leave it till morning, you'll have lost that 10 minutes.

Speak your mind

Why is it that when a man gives his opinion, he's strong and forthright, but when a woman does the same thing, she's a bitch?

BETTE DAVIS, ACTRESS

What would you do if your boss asked you to do a demeaning task, or if a man shoved you aside on a crowded bus, causing you to drop your bags? If you're like many women, you'd swallow your angry feelings rather than risk embarrassment by losing your temper.

However, think about the times you have spoken up for yourself or for others; using your anger constructively to underscore a point almost always changes things for the better. This is not to say that screaming and yelling will solve problems. Anger is an emotion that needs to be acted upon, not necessarily acted out. And, anger can help you to set limits, say no to unreasonable demands, and meet needs you'd have otherwise ignored. To better cope with everyday conflicts, keep these tips in mind:

Breathe easy If you feel as if you're really going to explode, take two or three very deep breaths, and then count to 10. Slowly and intentionally wipe away your angry expression by clenching and relaxing your jaw, forehead and mouth. These actions will help stop you – or at least slow you down – when you think you're going to say something rash.

Aim for compromise Common ground is easier to achieve than victory.

Get to the point Even if someone has rubbed you up the wrong way, try to sell a constructive solution.

Be straight Say what you feel in a simple, polite and direct way.

Redirect your energy Doing something physical, such as taking a walk around the block or doing a fast-paced 20 minutes on a treadmill, can help you use up the adrenaline in your bloodstream. Kicking a cardboard box around the room or pounding some plasticine can also help to calm you in an emergency.

 HEAL YOUR ANGRY PAST. Practise forgiveness. A grudge left to simmer can provide just enough irritation to maintain hair-trigger anger. Refusing to cling to resentment can provide long-term relief from your own negative emotions.

Know when to stop

Stop when you're hot.

ERNEST HEMINGWAY, AUTHOR

In other words, learn to pack it in gracefully at a point when you've achieved something, rather than in the middle of a problem. It's nearly always easier to return to it later.

Learning how to shut your workday attitudes and activities off, and move into the next phase of your day – perhaps picking up children from school and taking them home, or going out with friends – can help you get more enjoyment from each day. Set yourself a knocking-off time – whether it's 3 o'clock, 5 o'clock or 7 o'clock – when you will say, firmly, 'That's enough. I've done the best I could today. It's now over, I'm moving on'. Make a point of clearing up your desk as much as possible, so you don't leave with the depressing vision of an overwhelming mess to deal with the next day. Make a brief list of the most important things you have to do the next day, and put out the papers and files you need for that job so you feel you'll have a head start. Then leave.

Depending on how you travel to work – by car, bus, train or foot – make this time one of positive mental transition between work and home. If you have a longer commute, use the time for small, undemanding tasks such as list-making or for a pleasant interlude of reading or listening to music. Even if you only have 15 minutes, get into the habit of using that time to wind down and do nothing at all, just breathe deeply, organise your thoughts and consciously distance yourself from work worries. This is especially helpful when you're going home to children, giving you the chance to withstand the onslaught of their news, complaints and needs. Some mums even take the long route home on particularly harrowing days to try to get rid of tension before they see their children.

 CUT YOUR LOSSES. If you've put a huge amount of effort into something – a relationship, a fundraiser or a work project – for little or no return, set a time limit for results, and then change direction and put your energy into something else.

Planning essentials
The resume

What would happen if you got fired or retrenched today? Or, if you're presently working for yourself from home, what would happen if you saw a job advertised in the paper that looked interesting? If you have an up-to-date resume, you can act swiftly if necessary. Here's how:

Collate backup materials The resume itself is one thing, but being proactive in pursuing your work life means keeping orderly records of other relevant items, e.g. references, employment and tax records, and certificates of achievement. Keep an up-to-date portfolio of your best work.

Write and design a professional resume As a general rule, a title sheet should contain personal details (name, address, qualifications, perhaps a photograph of yourself). You might also want to include a personal mission statement, detailing your career objectives and personal strengths. This should be followed by your professional experience in chronological order, with the most recent position listed foremost. For each position held, give the job title, the commencement and leaving dates, and a brief summary of your key responsibilities and achievements within that role. Point form presentation is preferable as it is easier to read.

Keep a diary of accomplishments How much money did your initiative actually save the company? How many products did you help sell? How many people reported to you? Remember to ask yourself the Five Ws: Who? What? When? Where? and Why? By keeping specific records that prove your ability, you'll be well prepared for your next job interview.

Be prepared It's a jungle out there. Corporate upheavals mean that an unplanned job change is likely to be forced upon you at least once in your working life. Aim to have a nest egg in the bank that will tide you over for four to six months unemployment, or to fill the gap until the first cheque arrives from your new employer.

Get professional help There are many human resources consultants who will charge a small fee to help you prepare and polish a resume – it is money well spent.

The list

I would be lost without my lists. A daily to-do list has to be the best time saver there is. It gives you the chance to look at what you need (or at least would like) to get done that day, and put it in order of priority, giving your day a good start with a clear direction. Even if you only manage to tick off one item, at least you've done *something*, avoiding that thankless feeling of having been incredibly busy all day, but having nothing to show for it. A daily list helps you focus, clearing the mental clutter that crowds in and distracts you. It's particularly important when your tasks are small, relentless, domestic ones. Simply writing down, 'water garden', 'take back videos', 'stack boxes in cellar', makes the tasks achievable, and they lose their bugbear status. Here are some good tips to remember with list making:

Prioritise Number the tasks from the most to the least important to achieve. Set priorities based on importance, not just urgency.

Break large tasks into several smaller segments This way you can actually manage to tick off a couple and keep yourself motivated rather than feeling overwhelmed.

Estimate time It is a good idea to note how much time you think each task will take.

Be realistic There will be plenty of days when you don't get everything done. Instead of chastising yourself for not finishing every item on your list, congratulate yourself for being productive enough to manage what you have done, and move the rest to another day.

Keep your lists simple Texaco Chief Executive Peter Bijur is quoted as saying, 'As soon as you introduce complexity, the more difficult it is to operate'. Not only are two- or three-page lists too daunting, but you actually waste time writing them.

Make lists 'leak proof' Include every activity required for a particular project. For example, if your list doesn't include all the people you have to telephone that day, your mind still has to remember some of them.

Is it a could-do or a must-do task? In other words, don't get sidetracked with things that don't contribute to your goals for that day.

Write a don't-do list as well as a to-do one This should include any tasks you can give to someone else, anything that you do just to please others, and any job whose completion really doesn't matter much. Ask yourself, 'What's the worst that can happen if I don't do this?' If the answer is 'not much' – don't do it.

My second favourite household chore is ironing. My first being hitting my head on the top bunk bed until I faint.

ERMA BOMBECK, WRITER AND HUMORIST

Make home life sweeter

Welcome yourself home

Home is any four walls that enclose the right people.

HELEN ROWLAND, AUTHOR

There's nothing like entering your own front drive or path and feeling calm and happy to be home. Take a few tips from real estate agents who know exactly what makes a home feel welcoming and comfortable:

Plant perennials instead of annuals in the garden They establish themselves more quickly, grow more densely, and spread every year, with a minimum of fuss.

Keep the garbage bins out of sight If you haven't got a side path, build a simple box or lattice screen for them to sit behind.

Trim shrubs and branches around pathway and entrance It will stop you from feeling as though it's a struggle to get in the door. Also prune tree branches that touch the house.

Keep the paths swept If you have leaves or flowers dropping from trees, they can become slippery when wet and become a hazard.

Install decent outside lighting It is very important to do this over paths and steps.

Train your children Get them to place their shoes neatly at the door and hang their coats and hats on designated racks.

Keep things out of the way If you have animals, place food and water bowls in a spot that's out of the way of doors and paths. Keep the area clean.

Keep the garden neat Hang any hoses up neatly, or roll them over a hose wheel.

Hire a gardener They can do heavy work, such as pruning and lopping.

 HAVE POTS OF ANNUALS NEAR YOUR FRONT DOOR. That way you can enjoy their colour and variety without having to overhaul whole garden beds. Marigolds, pansies and zinnias all grow easily from seed and are very undemanding, only requiring you to pull off dead blooms as you walk past.

Create a relaxed bedroom

A rumpled, smelly bed is not conducive to sound sleep. Waking up in a messy room is also not a good way to start the day. Here's how to turn your bedroom into a haven:

Invest in good quality reading lamps They cast a warm and inviting, yet strong glow.

Keep just one book or magazine by your bed Big piles of reading material that you need to catch up on are draining to look at.

Don't store items under beds or on top of wardrobes It results in a heavy, burdened feeling to the room.

Treat yourself Always keep a vase of fresh flowers – even just a few leafy sprigs – on your dressing table or bureau.

Tidy up Quickly fluffing up the covers, opening a window, shutting drawers and bundling dirty clothes into the laundry basket will only take a scant minute in the morning, but will make all the difference to how you feel when you walk back into the bedroom at the end of a hard day.

Don't keep electrical equipment in your bedroom An electric clock radio next to the bed can cause disturbed sleep patterns; keeping a television or computer in the bedroom can make you anxious by reminding you of work, as well as adding electrical energy to the room that may compromise your ability both to relax and sleep.

USE SPACE BAGS (from hardware shops) to store winter blankets or doonas, and out-of-season clothes – pushing all the leftover air out of the bag reduces the amount of storage space needed.

Survive the school fete

Just when I think I can sit down with a book and a glass of wine, I fish a crumpled note out of the bottom of someone's school bag that tells me there's a cake stall the next day. When I've stopped screaming, out comes Nanna's old china mixing bowl and I start making my super-easy, never-fail chocolate brownies. Here's the recipe:

150 g (5 oz) butter, chopped

300 g (10 oz) dark chocolate, chopped coarsely

300 g (10 oz) firmly packed brown sugar

4 eggs

1 cup plain flour

$^1\!/_2$ cup sour cream

$^1\!/_2$ cup toasted walnuts, chopped coarsely

Preheat the oven to moderate (180°C/350°F).

Line the base and sides of a 20 cm × 30 cm (8" × 12") slice tin with baking paper.

Combine butter and chocolate in a medium saucepan.

Stir over a low heat until chocolate is just melted.

Transfer the chocolate mixture to a medium bowl and stir in the sugar.

Stir the lightly beaten eggs into the chocolate mixture, then the sifted flour, sour cream and walnuts.

Spread the mixture into the prepared pan.

Bake, uncovered, for about 30 minutes.

Cool in pan.

Next morning, cut brownie into 16 or 20 pieces, pop on a paper plate or into a gift box for child to take to school.

USE DISPOSABLE CONTAINERS. Don't use Tupperware or a china plate – you'll never get it back.

Resort to clichés

*Life is a grindstone. But whether it wears you down
or polishes you up is up to you.*

CAVETT ROBERT, AUTHOR

In the midst of negotiation, when bargaining, bribery and calm, logical discussion
have all failed, every mother knows that there are certain proverbs and phrases
whose time-honoured power can always be relied upon:

You can't have your cake and eat it too.

Where there's a will, there's a way.

First come, first served.

How do you know if you haven't tried it?

Eavesdroppers never hear any good of themselves.

Just wait till your father comes home.

Because it's good for you.

Some day you'll be grateful to me.

Think of all the starving children in … (currently miserable country).

A stitch in time saves nine.

The wind will change and you'll stay like that.

Waste not, want not.

Always wear clean underwear in case you get run over.

Better late than never.

Two heads are better than one.

(And best of all) Because I said so.

 DON'T UNDERESTIMATE CLICHÉS. They can bring order and comfort, or, at least,
a fleeting illusion of being in control.

Make manners count

It takes a Herculean amount of strength and patience – which I do not possess – to instil table manners in children, yet it's not possible to live together without them. To paraphrase John Lennon, here's what 'gets me through the meal':

Avoid clams or oysters 'What's this wiggly bit, Mum?' 'Of course you eat the head part.' Fat foods like artichokes, lobster and whitebait only in the presence of consenting adults.

Don't argue It's unkind to the digestion. If you want to argue about something, leave the table. (And that also goes for adults who gather around debating the Middle East and our trade deficit.)

Don't cough, sneeze, burp, belch or fart No dirty jokes, either. (Did I happen to mention I have two boys?) For that matter, adults can discuss diets, allergies and their recent hospital stays another time, too.

Don't be a Great Big Bore Don't show off, raise your voice, thump your fist, monopolise conversation or talk exclusively to one other person. No one likes to feel left out.

Don't fidget That includes, glass twirling, standing cutlery up on end, touching your plate to see if it's hot, nail picking, head scratching, drawing imaginary lines on the tablecloth, crumbling your bread into shapes, or rocking to-and-fro on your chair.

Don't be a pig Don't put too much food onto your plate – you can always come back for seconds. Don't put great chunks of food into your mouth, either – apart from looking revolting, you run the risk of choking. Eating quickly is bad manners, too – try to match your speed of eating with the others at the table so you all finish together.

Turn the TV off during mealtimes Same goes for videos, mobile phones, Walkmans and computer games.

 SAY THANK YOU. Always thank the person who's made the meal for you. It's pretty boring to have to wash, cook, iron, clean and put away dishes day after relentless day. A bit of appreciation goes a long way.

Don't take TV too seriously

Complete this phrase: 'Here's a story, about a lovely lady, who was bringing up three very lovely girls. All of them had hair of gold, like their mother . . .' What? You don't remember the theme song to *The Brady Bunch*, the seventies sitcom about Marcia, Greg, Peter, Jan, Cindy and Bobby which has been run and re-run zillions of times? All right, then, I'll give you an easier one. Name one show besides *I Dream of Jeannie* that Larry Hagman (Jeannie's Master) starred in. (All answers are below, but no peeking.) Oh, come ON. Here's one you can't possibly get wrong. What did Fred Flintstone, the cartoon caveman, call his pet?

Now I haven't dredged all this stuff up from any encyclopedia of television trivia. All the answers to these questions are crammed inside my head, ready to burst out at the slightest invitation. This should give you an idea of how much television I watched as a kid. I can tell you the name of Samantha's little girl in *Bewitched*, as well as the name of the boat which was shipwrecked on *Gilligan's Island*. Go ahead and ask me who was the host of the kids' quiz show, *It's Academic*. No problem. And I can sing the theme songs for *The Addams Family*, *The Munsters*, *Mission Impossible*, *M*A*S*H* . . . scary, isn't it?

Clearly, I was a TV junkie. And yet despite all those hours spent in front of that flickering black and white screen (I'm really dating myself now) somehow I turned out to be a more or less well-adjusted person (who just happens to know what Thurston Howell III called his wife). And my case is probably not a fluke. While television may indeed be a large waste of time – and there's plenty of evidence to show that it reduces fitness levels, gives young people unrealistic or potentially violent images, and force-feeds consumers products they don't really need – I think there are also some positives. For one thing, viewing quality television can be illuminating and reassuring. For another, watching a silly soap or rubbishy quiz show can sometimes be just the ticket for relaxing and unwinding.

 ANSWERS: '. . . the youngest one in curls. It's a story about a man named Brady, who was busy with three boys of his own. They were four men, living all together, yet they were all alone.'; *Dallas*; Dino; Tabitha; the *S.S. Minnow*; Andrew Harwood; Lovie.

50

Adolescence, anyone?

One of the most difficult things for loving, bewildered parents to get through their thick skulls is that their teenagers are, for the most part, quite happy underneath all their moody, surly behaviour. If you think you can fix things and 'make it better' for your little treasure, think again. Teenagers would rather be miserable doing what *they* choose than what *you* want them to do. Another thing: adolescence strikes (and that is the right word) very suddenly and with breathtaking strength. At our house, it seemed that one day I had two adorable cuddly boys in flannelette pyjamas, bounding on to the bed on a Sunday morning and the next I had a zoo filled with noisy, feral animals, slamming doors, horrible smells emanating from bedrooms, and furious insults ('Oh, *her*! What would she know?'). If it helps, I have learnt a few things that you won't necessarily read in books:

They don't hate you, even if they say they do They may feel completely bored by what you have to say, not to mention condescendingly pitying towards you for your lack of fashion sense, lack of brain, lack of cool – but they really don't hate you.

All teenagers lie I was heartbroken when Edward, my eldest, first lied to me, and proceeded to have a sombre talk with him about always telling the truth, trusting each other, etc. 'Don't worry, Mum, all the kids lie to their parents, I just wanted to see what you'd do', he said cheerfully.

Teenagers stick together This is part of the behaviour that sees them catch the same bus, walk in clumps and keep in constant touch via the telephone. You have the best chance of getting an answer or a conversation if no friends are around.

My sympathies are with the parents, actually. Adolescence is a difficult period, but completely normal and, except in unusual circumstances, approaching your offspring with too much understanding, empathy and tolerance just ends up excusing lousy behaviour. With rare exceptions, I think shifting responsibility from the parent to the child is a recipe for disaster. Instead, give your kids limited freedom, limited money, a strong code of behaviour and absolutely masses of love.

 YOU CAN NEVER GIVE YOUR CHILD TOO MUCH LOVE. Don't just give them peck-on-the-cheek-goodnight love, give them the big-compliment-always-interested-bear-hug type of love. Tell them how gorgeous and clever and capable they are every single day. Tell them even when you are ringing up the motor mechanic for a quote on the dinged fender or looking at his or her latest report.

Motherhood is not for the faint-hearted. Frogs, skinned knees and the insults of teenage girls are not meant for the wimpy.

DANIELLE STEELE

Treat yourself to lovely linen

Let's go to that house, for the linen looks white and smells of lavender and I long to be in a pair of sheets that smell so.

IZAAK WALTON, 16th CENTURY AUTHOR OF *THE COMPLEAT ANGLER*

An often-neglected item in many households is linen. Sheets and towels frequently get pulled out and shoved back any old which way. Here's how to get your linens in order:

Sheets Considering a third of our lives is spent in bed, it makes sense to invest in the most attractive, best quality sheets and bedding you can afford. You should have two sets of sheets and pillowcases per bed, which allows you to have one in the wash and one on the bed.

Blankets and doonas Keep at least one warm winter blanket and one lighter or cotton blanket per bed. If you don't own a doona or quilt, plan on stocking a couple of extra blankets per bed.

Soft, thick towels These are luxurious to use as well as being practical – thick towels will last much longer than cheaper, thinner ones. You'll need a minimum of two per person in the household, plus two bath mats. Stock at least four small hand-towels for guests, and terry towelling facecloths according to the number of people who use them.

 USE A MATTRESS PROTECTOR. It will save your mattress from wear and tear and extend its life.

Organise your sewing kit

A stitch in time saves nine.

PROVERB

It's a waste of time and money to have to run to an expensive mending service or tailor for minor repairs. A prudently stocked sewing kit should contain:

needles in assorted sizes

thread in basic colours, such as black, white, and beige

thimble

needle threader (especially if your eyesight isn't what it used to be)

sharp scissors

extra buttons (all those extra buttons that come with new clothes should be automatically popped in)

safety pins (for temporary repairs until you can get around to fixing it properly)

iron-on patches (a must-have for instantly fixing knees-out and tears in school clothes)

 DON'T DELAY SEWING REPAIRS. It's disheartening to have piles of torn or stained clothing accumulating in your cupboards.

Enjoy your nest

My favourite therapy? Rearranging the furniture.

BETTY FRIEDAN, FEMINIST

I am the kind of person who actually enjoys planting petunias and painting outdoor furniture; someone who will elbow for the last leg of lamb in the butcher's window for her family. My favourite song is, 'What a Wonderful World', my desk calendar is the one made by Randall, my son, in kindergarten, with the picture stuck on upside down. My house has fairy lights in the tree outside the kitchen window, mint growing by the tap and two cats who live on the mantelpiece in winter. I love yellow roses, Willowware jugs and tapestry slippers.

Taking time for the small things that make a house a welcoming home – spreading an embroidered linen centrepiece on the dining table, arranging a bunch of flowers, placing some knick-knacks or photos in a new spot – is not to be dismissed as trivial. They are small, easily achievable steps towards making a little time for yourself and feeling a little more in control of your environment.

Make a list of all the simple things that make you happy, and surround yourself with more of them. They rarely have to be big or expensive. You can't put off being happy, waiting for some mythical perfect time and place where everything will be just right. Not only will you deprive yourself, but you will be doing other people – especially your children – a disservice. Being happy is a state of mind, a choice to behave a certain way that you adopt every single day, and it starts at home. If you surround yourself with things that inspire you and make you happy, then the people around you will be happier too.

SURROUND YOURSELF WITH BEAUTIFUL THINGS – sights, smells and textures that give you glimpses of pleasure.

Plan meals ahead

The statistics on sanity are that one out of every four women is suffering from some form of mental illness. Think of your three best friends. If they're OK, then it's you.

RITA MAE BROWN

My mother used to call it 'the arsenic hour'. It falls between 5 pm and 7 pm, when you're tired and running late, the kids are cranky and starving, and you need to get a decent meal on the table as quickly as possible. These ideas can help:

Have family favourites Identify a couple of very easy dinners that everyone likes and that rely mainly on non-perishable items that are always handy: pasta and pre-made sauce (plus grated cheese and a salad); pizza (frozen pizza base, bottled pasta sauce, any selection of meat, cheese and vegies); or fried rice (rice, canned and/or frozen vegetables, frozen ham or bacon).

Plan dinners for the week Then write a weekly shopping list.

Check out prepared meals and ingredients Cut and washed lettuce, peeled and quartered potatoes, and pre-seasoned, griller-ready chicken breasts all reduce food preparation time to virtually zero.

Everyone should help Even small children can clear and set the table or toss a salad. In addition to helping you, it gives them a sense of responsibility and can be a welcome distraction from how hungry they are.

Appoint a 'surprise chef' This idea comes from a friend with four teenagers and a full-time job. Every Friday night, each of the kids takes it in turns to decide what's for dinner, get extra ingredients if necessary, prepare the meal, and clean up afterwards. The menu served up by the youngest boy on his first night has become a favourite family story: green jelly, cocktail frankfurts and mashed potato, plus paper plates and cups, because he didn't want to have to wash up.

TURN YOUR ANSWERING MACHINE ON AT DINNERTIME. Even the quickest meal is a chance to reconnect with others, so don't let it be lost to interruptions.

Planning essentials
The noticeboard

If handled poorly, messages, written notes and instructions between members of the family can be a major source of frustration and even disaster. In my household, everyone needs to communicate, but everyone is on different schedules! The best thing you can do is set up a noticeboard. Here's how to make it work:

Decide on one There are two main types of noticeboard: a whiteboard on which you can use magnetised buttons to display cards or newsletters, or which can be written on and erased (in which case, tie the eraser and pen to the side of the board so they don't disappear); or a cork or fabric-covered bulletin board (in which case, store tacks or pins in a container nearby). If buying a cork or fabric-covered model, stretch ribbon in a crosswise pattern to-and-fro and secure at the back. This way, you can slide larger items in that might be too heavy to be pinned up.

Go for big, bright and beautiful As a general rule, the bigger the noticeboard, the better. Make it user-friendly by picking one that you like to look at – a bright colour may add to your enjoyment.

Position, position, position Hang your noticeboard in a prominent place, close to a door that is used most often to go in and out of the house, e.g. next to the back door or in the kitchen. That way, you can easily grab letters to be mailed or check notes and incoming messages as you start and end the day. You might need to put it at a lower level if you have small children.

Divide and conquer The best system I have come up with entails dividing the noticeboard into four sections, naming one for each of us, then pinning our mail, notes, party invitations, and phone messages under our names.

Display vital information The family noticeboard is a prime spot to keep on permanent display a sheet listing important details, e.g. emergency phone numbers for the fire brigade, ambulance, vet, doctor or dentist, and everyone's mobile numbers.

Keep it clear Get into the habit of pruning your noticeboard regularly (a great use for one of those 10-minute snippets of time!) and update or toss out all the little scraps of paper, school notices and permission slips as soon as they are out of date.

The home magazines

My secret vice is homemaker magazines, so much so that my husband calls them 'Pamela's Porn'. On a scale of pigsty to presentable, my house veers towards the pigsty end, which is probably why I find it so soothing to look at photographs of beautiful gardens and inviting verandahs. Still, your house isn't just a roof over your head. If you've already taken the big steps to unclutter much of your home environment – the kitchen, the cupboards and the wardrobe – it's time to create a home environment that feeds your spirit and is a well-deserved retreat from the world. Homemaker magazines are a great place to start getting ideas. Here's how:

Look at the big picture Naturally, any home renovation is dependent on your budget (or lack of it), but the first step is to make some decisions about your home's design, how it flows, its functionality and ease of maintenance. Simple changes, such as converting an existing window into a pair of French doors leading out to the garden, or putting a skylight in a kitchen or bathroom, can make a huge difference in making your home more comfortable as well as increasing its value.

Do it yourself Homemaker magazines are also a great source of time- and cost-saving information on fix-it-yourself methods for common household predicaments, such as unclogging sinks and tubs, fixing dripping taps, and blocked toilets.

Consider the placement of furniture and ornaments in your home Do you find that people regularly walk into a corner table, or trip over a rug? Certain floor plans seem to work better than others, perhaps creating better traffic flow, allowing more light into a room, or just putting things where they're more convenient to reach. On a more subtle level, the ancient Chinese art of feng shui tells us that how people interact with the building structure itself as well as with the items inside that building, will affect their energy levels. Some of the main feng shui rules include: avoiding sharp angles in favour of rounded shapes; incorporating natural elements and materials wherever possible; using some warm colours or candles in every room (to represent fire and the related emotions of love and passion); placing lights in dark corners; and bringing running water into the house in the form of a fish tank or fountain (both for a calming effect and to encourage prosperity).

Move things around If a room seems stagnant or cold, move the furniture, put away some ornaments and bring out new ones, or roll up the rugs for a change.

The only place where success comes before work is in the dictionary.

VIDAL SASSOON, HAIRDRESSER

Getting things done

Morning madness

Most mums would agree that getting everyone up and out the door in the morning is, at best, a challenge and at worst, a flurry of slaps, tears, spilled food and slammed doors. Even the most hectic days work out better than expected if they start well. These ideas will help:

Keep things handy Put a hatstand in the hallway to keep everyone's hats and umbrellas together. Fill a lidded jar with change and keep it there for school lunches, last-minute expenses, tolls, meters and fares.

Set your alarm clock 15 minutes early Get up when it goes off, rather than waiting. Even if you don't need those extra 15 minutes for a last-minute emergency, it makes you much more relaxed to know that they're there.

Give everyone jobs that they have to do For example, taking their own plates to the sink, feeding pets.

Choose easy-to-prepare, easy-to-eat breakfasts for weekdays For example, cereal, muesli, porridge with milk, yoghurt and fruit, or baked beans on toast. Encourage older children to make their own breakfast. For younger children who are attending daycare or kindergarten, the best policy is to regard lunch as their major meal of the day. Passing the responsibility to the caregiver in this way takes the pressure off you for breakfast and dinner.

Get kids moving With kids, money is a great incentive. Each week, I put five $1 coins in two jars, one for each son. If one son is slow and holds everyone else up, I take a coin out of his jar. They get what's left in their jar at the end of the week.

Make lunch in advance Make a week's worth of sandwiches in one evening and freeze them (no egg or mayonnaise, though).

Slow and steady wins the race Make an effort to move and talk in a very relaxed manner in the mornings. Drive within the speed limit; pause before you reply to a question; let the phone ring a few times before you answer it. Start out 10 minutes early instead of waiting until the last possible moment. You won't have to rush, and you'll be less stressed.

DO AS MUCH AS POSSIBLE THE NIGHT BEFORE. Set out clothes, car keys, schoolbags and briefcases; iron clothes; and make lunches and put them in the fridge. You'll start your day feeling less frazzled and more in command.

Make-up shake-up

*I don't have time to put on lipstick every morning.
I need that time to clean my rifle.*

HENRIETTE MANTEL, FEMINIST AND COMEDIENNE

You can slice many valuable minutes off your morning routine by following this advice:

Adopt the less-is-more rule Instead of a complicated regime of foundation, cover stick, powder and blush, opt for a quick once-over with an all-in-one tinted moisturiser and sunblock product, followed by a lick of mascara and a touch of lipstick.

Choose cosmetic colours that coordinate with each other For example, shades of pink or brown rather than cluttering up your make-up box or bag with eye shadows and lipsticks that only go with one particular outfit.

Stop bathroom congestion Keep all your cosmetics and hair-styling preparations in your bedroom, or near where you will be getting dressed, rather than in the bathroom, thus avoiding congestion when someone else is in there having a shower or cleaning their teeth.

 GET A SIMPLE, WELL-CUT HAIRSTYLE that is easy to maintain and, preferably, that can dry naturally rather than require a full blow-dry each morning.

Get a head start

Some days it seems all I've managed to do is have a sip of coffee and pick a few dead leaves off my geranium plant on the kitchen windowsill, and suddenly it's five o'clock. Starting your day in a slow and circuitous way – letting phone calls or drop-in visitors rob your time, fretting over what to do first or getting caught up with lots of fussy little jobs before you start your 'real' work – can then set the tone for the rest of the day. The way you feel at the end of the day is tied directly to your success in focussing on that day's top priority. Here are some tips for getting off to a good start:

Every night, make a to-do list for the next day Check it, number the tasks in order of priority, and then rewrite it before leaving it where you'll see it first thing in the morning, for example, on your computer screen or next to your place at the breakfast table. This works on a subconscious level: you'll think about it that evening and visualise yourself tackling those tasks in that order.

Always set aside enough time to get yourself ready Shower, dress and eat breakfast.

Check email and phone messages first thing But only deal with urgent ones straightaway. Put non-essential messages to one side for later.

Discourage time wasters If you work in an office where a certain amount of sociable behaviour is expected, you need to manage those people who want to chat, however briefly. Rather than sit and talk, say, 'I'm just going downstairs to drop off this report, but you can tell me on the way if you like'. That way your work gets done at the same pace, and you won't be thought of as stand-offish or disinterested.

Ask for help If you're stewing over a project you don't understand and just can't seem to get it underway, ask for help to move things along. If you're experiencing real difficulties, find a mentor or someone you can trust to advise you. All too often we feel as if we should do everything ourselves and that asking for help is a sign of failure. It's actually a sign of confidence and success.

 START EACH DAY ON THE RIGHT FOOTING. Begin with a small ritual that works for you. It could be using a special cup for your tea, or reading an inspirational quote on a page-a-day calendar, or a favourite cartoon strip in the morning newspaper. Humour, beauty and poetry add spice and meaning to our lives.

Make your commute count

It is the moment that you think you can't, that you can.

CELINE DION, SINGER

If you manage it correctly, your commuting time can be a gift that helps you to plan and enjoy your day. Here are some ideas to try:

Catch up on work If you catch a train or bus, rather than just sitting and staring into space for anything up to an hour each day, work on your laptop computer. Prepare to send memos and emails, and catch up on paperwork; jot down notes and ideas on a notepad. If you're in a car, or on a train, bus or plane, you can also listen to educational audio cassettes or CDs while you travel – turn travel time into learning time.

Take time-out You certainly don't have to work, either. A commute can be just the right length of time for listening to music, motivational tapes or talking books on a walkman; reading; doing a crossword; or even sewing.

Get some exercise Depending on how far you live from your workplace, consider ditching public transport, and walking or jogging to work instead. Not only will this provide much-needed exercise, fresh air, and a chance to burn off pent-up energy if you have a sedentary job, it's also a great way to get your grey matter into gear.

 GET OUT OF THAT CHAIR. A 15-minute spin around the block is all it takes to blow the cobwebs away and help reorganise your thoughts.

Avoid telephone traps

In hell, all the messages you ever left on other people's answering machines will be played back to you.

JUDY HORACEK, COMEDIENNE

The summer my son Edward turned 13, we put in another phone line: 'Yes!' said all his friends, and proceeded to keep *both* lines busy. Teenagers are a prime example of how not to use the telephone, yet plenty of adults aren't much better. These ideas will make sure your phone is a help, not a hindrance:

Keep a minute timer near the phone It will remind you to be brief. You can also be sneaky and set the bell if your caller isn't getting the hint.

Practise polite brush-offs for non-essential calls Try 'I can't talk for long', or, 'I've got someone coming in right now for an appointment', so nobody loses face. Or start your conversation with something like, 'Nice to talk to you, but I'm just on my way out – perhaps I could call you back tonight?' Only in dire emergencies should anyone demand your attention when you don't want to give it.

Get rid of cold callers One of my pet peeves is when the phone rings as I'm cooking dinner and somebody starts trying to either sell me someting, or ask me questions for a survey. Over a year, it's hours of your time that's being wasted.

Screen calls Use your answering machine or voicemail while you're trying to concentrate on an important task, but be discreet. No one likes talking away on a message tape only to have you finally pick up because you've decided you do want to talk to them after all!

Get a cordless telephone You can stir the bolognese sauce, let the cat out, answer the front door and run a child's bath, all during the same conversation. And you can do all sorts of things while you're on hold.

Designate a message centre It should be the first place everyone checks for messages and mail – both at home and at work.

 MAKE AND RETURN PHONE CALLS AT A SET TIME. Set aside a portion of your day as telephone time. Let people know that this is the best time to reach you by phone and they won't bother you as much during the rest of the day.

Every mother is a working mother.
The only difference is that some
of them get paid for it.

MARGUERITE KELLY, AUTHOR

Meetings, schmeetings

One of my favourite clients, Ross, is famous for his super-short meetings. He is always on time, he doesn't serve tea or coffee, he always has an agenda ready, and never takes calls while you're there. I've been in and out of his office in 15 minutes flat, with a clear run at the whole morning ahead of me. He admits that several business associates have found his approach confronting, even rude, but for anyone wanting to be better organised, managing meetings has to be a prime target. These ideas will help:

Ask yourself if it's absolutely necessary to go If the goal can be achieved via email, telephone or fax, so much the better. Have the confidence not to attend if you're only going to 'be seen'.

If it's your meeting, have an agenda – three to four points maximum Do the big things first, the small things second. Schedule time blocks for each item to be discussed.

Bring all necessary documents If you're attending someone else's meeting, have all the papers or documents they'll want to see.

Decide in advance when the meeting will start and finish Let participants know this information before the meeting begins.

Arrive on time and start on time, even if everyone isn't there Keep track of time. Comments such as, 'We only have 30 minutes left', help keep people focussed. Go as soon as the main business is concluded. It's extraordinary how many people have difficulty being the first to get up, say thank you and go. Are they worried that they'll be talked about when they're gone?

Be alert for detours It's easy to get sidetracked and wind up debating something else. Stick to the agenda; if necessary, suggest a follow-up call or meeting to discuss the other matter.

 STAND UP. A study in *Psychology Today* compared meetings at which everyone stood, with sit-down conferences where the same subjects were discussed. The decisions made in the stand-up meetings were just as accurate as the sit-down versions, and took half as long to reach.

Using technology

It is not the strongest of the species that survives, nor the most intelligent. It is the one that is most adaptable to change.

CHARLES DARWIN, SCIENTIST AND AUTHOR

Thanks to email and the Internet, we have a brand new way of keeping in touch and finding information. If you are a novice, enrol in an Internet training session. Here's what you need to know to use the Internet to your advantage:

Be selective and succinct Think about who you give your email address to. Remember, long messages are less likely to be read by busy people.

Don't use capitals This is like shouting in cyberspace, and is very rude.

Always include a headline Subject lines like, 'Hi from me' are a waste of time, having to be reopened and checked before being deleted.

Answer quickly One of email's greatest advantages is to cut down on response time. If you've been sent a report, for example, a three-word email, 'Received, with thanks', eliminates the need for a phone call.

Count to 10 The downside about email's speediness is that it's very easy to fire off a furious response. By all means, write your reply – but save it in your drafts file and re-read it before deciding whether you'll send it.

Don't routinely forward jokes Only send such material to people you know will appreciate it, and who have the time to read it.

Beware the company server Most companies have procedures in place to check and block incoming and circulating emails. The contents of emails can constitute grounds for discrimination, harassment and other forms of corporate misconduct.

Think Internet first Any of the following tasks can also be done on the Internet, saving you precious time: buying books, gifts, theatre tickets, clothes; checking movie times, sports results and weather; downloading application forms; learning languages;paying bills; booking holidays; searching for property.

Don't forsake all human contact Remember that people like to talk to each other and face-to-face meetings are much more effective for certain aspects of business.

 USE TECHNOLOGY TO YOUR ADVANTAGE. It should make life easier, not harder.

Handle interruptions

Can't finish one thing before something else comes up? It's unrealistic to plan a completely interruption-free day. However, you can learn to be far more ruthless in determining what is and what isn't an important or necessary interruption:

Ask if it can wait Say your boss has interrupted you with a job that needs to be done straightaway. Rather than drop everything, first say, 'These are the other jobs I'm working on right now. Please take just a moment to tell me whether any of these are more important than this new one. If so, I'll have to do them first'. The other person will often step back and say that the task can wait – at least until you've finished several others.

Screen phone calls Use your voicemail or answering machine to separate essential from non-essential calls. Discipline yourself to finish what you're doing wherever possible, rather than dropping everything to return a call or email.

See if there's a pattern Quite often – especially in an office – there is one person who interrupts you far more often than others. It may be because they're bored or under-employed, maybe they've found you to be a quick way to get answers to questions they would otherwise have to spend time on, or perhaps they're just lonely and looking for recognition. Keep a list of interruptions in your day, and you'll quickly see whether there is a particular pattern, such as a salesperson pestering you, or a subordinate constantly asking for further instructions.

Put papers on your office guest chair This keeps people from popping in and having a chat for no reason.

GIVE THOROUGH INSTRUCTIONS. Explain to a colleague how you want a task done – otherwise they'll be constantly pestering you, wanting more information.

Do two things at once

*Whatever women do they must do twice as well as men
to be thought half as good. Luckily, this is not difficult.*

CHARLOTTE WHITTON, CANADIAN POLITICIAN

The secret to feeling better organised around the home is to do other small tasks while waiting for big things to finish, like cooking or washing. For instance, while watching TV, you could also be putting photos in albums, riding an exercise bike, folding the washing, doing small sewing repairs such as putting on buttons or giving yourself a manicure. There are endless ideas – here are just a few:

Add things to your shopping list

Fill the kettle

Take out any rubbish

Stack the dishwasher, or quickly wash dirty dishes as you go.

Switch on the sprinkler or water the pot plants.

Prepare kids' lunches for the next day.

Check and toss out leftovers in the fridge.

Plug in your mobile to recharge.

Make a quick phone call.

FILL IN GAPS. Those little left-over snatches of time when you're kept waiting for an appointment, delayed in traffic or commuting to-and-from work, can be used more effectively. Listen to a walkman, pop a talking book in the car's cassette player, learn a foreign language, write thankyou cards, read a magazine or plan a menu.

Taking it on the road

He who would travel happily and see where he is going must travel light.

ANTOINE DE SAINT-EXUPERY, AUTHOR

Whether you're a regular business traveller, or just go away on the odd weekend, being a savvy packer can save time and reduce stress. Here's what to remember:

Make sure your suitcase is in good condition and accessible Try to pack one that you can carry on the plane with you to save time.

Leave essentials in your case Buy travel-size bottles of favourite toiletries and pack underwear, pantyhose, nightwear, fold-up umbrella, travel hairdryer, emergency medical kit, and zip-lock plastic bags for holding things like leaky bottles. That way, you can go at a moment's notice.

Record important details You should write down relevant phone numbers, addresses, and flight numbers and times, either in your address book or electronic organiser and keep it in your carry-on luggage. If you're travelling overseas, particularly through any troubled areas, find out contact details for embassies. Prepare an itinerary and list the details of people you are seeing, in order of when you will be meeting them. If there's time, get hold of a street directory and work out directions before you arrive.

Have extra cash on hand Take at least an extra $100 in a zipped pocket in your bag for unforeseen emergencies. Having to find an ATM in a strange city in the early hours of the morning is inconvenient and stressful.

Carry at least one internationally accepted credit card Sign up for Credit Card Sentinel, or similar, which provides you with a 24-hour cancellation service anywhere in the world in case of loss or theft.

Make sure you can be contacted Most mobile phones offer an option for voicemail that can be accessed anywhere in the world via a security code.

 BE SAFETY CONSCIOUS. Laptop computers and phones are regularly stolen while their owner pays for coffee in an airport lounge. Be discreet while speaking on a phone in a hotel or airport – you never know who is listening to your comments about where you are staying or who you are seeing.

Instead of thinking about where you are, think about where you want to be. It takes twenty years of hard work to become an overnight success.

DIANA RANKIN, AUTHOR

Do lunch

Men do lunch – women do errands.

CAR BUMPER STICKER

It's true – women are far more likely than men to pack a lunch and take it to work, so they'll have time to pick up the drycleaning or get something from the newsagent for a school project. Granted, the errands aren't going to disappear, but there is still plenty of opportunity for reconfiguring your precious lunchbreaks in life-enhancing ways:

Aim for balance Choose between enjoyable and productive lunches with good friends and work associates, and time-wasting ones. Aim for a healthy balance – say, one casual lunch with friends every week, a work-related one every fortnight.

Escape one day a week Find a place where you can have absolute calm and quiet. Whether you work at home or in the middle of the city, you can still find a church, a library or a park where you won't be disturbed.

Make phone calls Catch up with friends and family during lunchtime.

Exercise Take a brisk walk or go for a jog.

Read something Even if you have next to no time, you can still dip into a book of short stories, inspirational poetry or essays, or zip through a couple of magazine articles.

VISIT A MUSEUM OR ART GALLERY. Prowl through a craft shop or antique centre. This is not to be confused with shopping or spending money – it's about refreshing your mind with different sights and ideas.

Think long-term

Getting caught up in immediate work concerns and not spending enough time planning for the longer term can not only negatively affect your sense of happiness and satisfaction – because you feel as though you're not really moving forward – it can also make you vulnerable to business competition.

Putting together plans should involve looking at what you want on a weekly, monthly, and long-term basis. Set aside time to think carefully about what your goals are, and then break them down into sets of objectives, prioritise them, and create a schedule for achieving them. With every goal, ask yourself, 'Is this really what I want to do with my life?' Planning your time is not just about how much you can get done – it's about planning how you want to spend your life. Here's how:

Think about the 'big picture' What are the things that really make your heart sing? What do you want to experience in your work and home life? It's easy to lose sight of what's really important.

List specific objectives and goals Owning a home and/or car, spending more time with family and friends, and planning holidays are some obvious ones. Underneath each item, make a list of the specific actions you need to work through to achieve it, such as, 'Set up an automatic salary deduction every week to pay off mortgage faster'. Some goals, especially the ones like, 'Spend more time with family', will be harder to quantify (which is why they often never happen). Nail down simple but achievable actions, such as, 'Invite Mum to lunch'.

Lock it in Estimate time involved for each of the first few actions, and write them in your diary, to-do list or calendar, to get things moving. For example, make that appointment with the accountant for next week.

Review your progress Every month, get out your long-term plan, tick off tasks and set new ones that lead you closer to your goals. Some months you may achieve several tasks, other months only one, but always give yourself credit for how far you've come.

KNOW YOUR GOALS. Some people never stop to question why they're doing the job they do. To what end are you working so hard? Are you on the career track you really want? If not, what do you want to be doing and how can you make it possible? One study of 8000 people found that an essential key to human happiness is loving your everyday profession. Do you love what you do?

Keep track of time

No matter how you juggle your schedule, the number of hours in the day will remain the same, and it's easy to underestimate how long something will take you to complete. Here's how to adjust your habits to buy more time for the things that matter most:

Have a safety net Always allocate yourself an extra five to ten minutes

Be conscious of how long you're spending on a task Practise jotting a start and finish time on your blotter or notepad, and adjust the rest of your schedule accordingly.

Try keeping a log or diary on yourself Seeing how much time you fritter away unnecessarily can be a real eye-opener. I did this when I started writing this book, breaking it up into time spent on unpaid home administrative tasks (e.g. going to the bank, post office, drycleaners and library); chores (e.g. shopping and cooking); paid work; time spent on myself (e.g. going to the hairdresser); goofing-off time (getting lost en route to my son's baseball game); and so on. After about 700 hours – nearly a month – I added up the hours and worked them out as percentages, and found I was spending an astonishing 35 per cent of my time on unpaid home administrative tasks. I decided that, in order to reach my goals of writing more, and spending time helping at my sons' schools, I either needed to delegate some of these tasks, or figure out more efficient ways of doing them, such as Internet banking.

 WEAR A WATCH. Being conscious of the pressure of time puts you in control of it.

Set deadlines

Very little is needed to make a happy life. It is all within yourself, in your way of thinking.

MARCUS AURELIUS, ROMAN PHILOSOPHER

My son Edward was dawdling over a school assignment, and I couldn't understand why he hadn't finished. The penny dropped when he complained that, 'The dumb teacher didn't explain it properly'. He'd succumbed to the paralysing fear many of us face: don't ask questions, it'll make you look stupid.

The first rule of working smarter is to clarify straightaway what is required of you and get all the information you need to get on with it, rather than waiting for the next meeting or class, in the hope that it will become clearer. These are other good tips:

Break it down Work out high and low priority aspects of the job. Ask yourself what is the most important aspect to be working on right now, and start on that.

Report regularly Touch base with the person you're doing the job for, whether it's your boss or a client. Knowing that they're keeping tabs on you is an incentive and also a backstop in case something unexpected happens.

Schedule concentration time Block out some time every day when you can't be disturbed except in an emergency. Use that time to tackle the next important task for which you have a close deadline. If someone interrupts you, you can politely reply, 'No, I'm in the middle of something right now, and I can't give you my full attention'.

Reward yourself Every time you make it past a section of the work required for your deadline, give yourself a little treat – buy a magazine, go out for a nice lunch, give yourself permission to enjoy a long, lazy Sunday morning lie-in.

Expect quality, rather than perfection Many people who have trouble meeting deadlines have the unrealistic idea that their work should be perfect.

 USE PARETO'S PRINCIPLE. It is a well-known term in management theory, that states that 80 per cent of your accomplishments come from 20 per cent of your efforts. So, think strategically – what 20 per cent of your work is the most valuable, to you and to your employer? Once you've identified it, try to focus the lion's share of your time and energy in that direction.

Planning essentials
The calendar

I live by the big calendar on the fridge. It has plenty of room per day for all the dates for the boys' school and sporting activities, plus I mark ahead of time when particular bills are due, which helps me save up for them, and I write in major personal appointments and birthdays. Choose the style that suits you best – large, small, desktop, fridge or a fold-out one to slip in your handbag or briefcase. As soon as
you agree to any appointment or activity, write it down on the calendar – or write yourself a note to jot it on the calendar when you get home.

Make a habit of looking at your calendar at the same time every day – for me, that's first thing in the morning, while I'm waiting for the kettle to boil for my much-needed cup of Irish Breakfast tea.

The diary

Keep track of appointments, due dates, deadlines and meetings in a diary. Choose the type you feel most comfortable using: this could be a Filofax type book, a week-at-a-glance desk diary or an electronic organiser; some people like to have a full page devoted to each day of the week, others find a compact system more suitable. I think diaries with separate sections for notes, telephone numbers and projects are far more useful than just appointment calendars. Here are some tips to make your diary work harder for you:

Keep your diary with you at all times Otherwise you end up writing things down on scraps of paper and the backs of old envelopes that get lost.

Write down everything that is a firm commitment Do not trust your memory! Writing it down also enables you to see activities in relation to one another.

Schedule in generous amounts of time Allow enough travelling time, for example, or time for finding a parking spot, or to accommodate unpredictable public transport.

Review your diary at the same time every day It's better to do it either first thing in the morning or last thing at night. This shouldn't take more than a few minutes, and it prevents nasty surprises.

Write everything in pencil!

Use only one diary Things tend to fall over if you have two or three, as you will invariably forget to transfer information from one to another.

Can you imagine a world without men?
No crime and lots of happy, fat women.

NICOLE HOLLANDER, WRITER

Health and fitness

Reclaim your fitness

I've been on a constant diet for the last two decades. I've lost a total of 789 pounds. By all accounts, I should be hanging from a charm bracelet.

ERMA BOMBECK, HUMORIST AND AUTHOR

If you're fit, you can function – if not, you'll find it even more difficult to get through what needs to be done. I go for a walk as soon as I get up; before I have time to think about it, I pull on a tracksuit and I'm out that door. If I wait till later in the day, it doesn't happen. Disciplining yourself to stick to a regular time is half the battle – if you're not a morning person, you might prefer a lunchtime jog, or a swim in the local pool on the weekend. Keep these ideas in mind:

Use stairs, not escalators or lifts It's nearly always only a flight or two.

Do two things at once Do leg lifts or knee bends while you're brushing your teeth. Stretch or walk around while you talk on a cordless phone.

Play with your kids Get out there and ride a bike or have a go on the swings. Walk up and down the sidelines while you watch them play football or netball.

Walk wherever possible Walk up the street to get milk or bread. Park and then walk to the theatre, school or office – apart from the exercise, it almost always saves time and money otherwise spent trying to get a 'good' parking spot.

Try Eastern-style exercise Even the most diehard couch potatoes can enjoy graceful practices such as yoga and tai chi that enhance physical and spiritual wellbeing.

Purchase exercise equipment Buy a stationary bike, treadmill or mini-trampoline so you can grab small snatches of exercise time at home.

Dance while you dust House cleaning can be a good aerobic workout if you put on dance music while you work.

 MANAGE STRESS. Even if you think you manage stress well, your body may be screaming for help. Insomnia, back pain, heartburn, headaches, loss of appetite (or feeling hungry all the time) and lowered sex drive are just a few of the physical symptoms of chronic stress.

Get instant energy

Your body creates energy from nutrients, oxygen and invigorating stimuli, such as fragrances. These natural mood and body boosters suit busy lives because they give you an instant lift and are so simple to do:

Massage your ears According to traditional Chinese medicine, stimulating acupressure points on your ears increases blood circulation, and thus energy. Vigorously rub your ears all over for about one minute. They should start to feel hot almost immediately, and you should feel more alert.

Take a power shower Sprinkle eucalyptus oil on the floor of your shower before stepping in. Stand under steaming hot water and rub your body with a loofah. The scent stimulates your brain while the hot water and the rub down increase blood flow, sending oxygen to your blood cells where it's transformed into energy.

Drink water Many people feel tired because they don't drink enough water. Their body fluids become thicker and move more sluggishly, slowing down circulation and impairing the chemical reactions in energy-producing cells.

Snack for long-term energy The best snacks provide a mix of protein, complex carbohydrates and fat, because the body metabolises them slowly. Smart snack choices include apple slices with peanut butter; multigrain toast with hummus or low-fat cheese; or plain low-fat yoghurt with a handful of chopped fresh fruit.

Wake up with a break Your body can only handle about 45 minutes of sitting without becoming fatigued. Get up and march around briskly for three to five minutes, or do some quick stretches or squats.

Make a splash Dip a facecloth in cold water and wet both the front and back of your neck. Then gargle with cold water for a couple of seconds. Your neck and throat are rich with sensitive nerves; by stimulating them with the cold water, you shock them into the 'fight-or-flight' reaction, which temporarily directs more blood towards your brain.

BREATHE FIRE. Sitting for long stretches of time causes carbon dioxide to build up in your blood, making you sleepy. The 'breath of fire' is a traditional yoga exercise that helps clear the lungs completely. First, breathe in deeply through your nose; then exhale using 15 to 20 short, sharp bursts, clenching your stomach muscles to really push out each burst. Repeat three times.

Walk your way to inner strength

A daily walk is not just an opportunity for exercise, it's a time to meditate, mull over the day's objectives, burn off a bad mood, and become more attuned to yourself. Here's how:

Start with stretches Before setting off, do a few fundamental stretches.

Breathe to the rhythm Synchronise your walking and breathing. A good rhythm to adopt is to breathe in through your nose while counting four steps – one, two, three, four – then breathe out through your mouth over the next four steps.

Engage your brain Time a chant or a mantra to each footfall, such as, 'I am here and I am clear' – pause – 'I am here and I am clear' – and so on. Two other good ones are, 'I can do this' – pause – 'I can do this', and, 'I am seeing, I am feeling, I am hearing'. You could say the thought or mantra out loud, or recite it to yourself in your mind.

Walk purposefully Hold your head up, relax your shoulders so they move with your torso as you walk – don't strain them back – and tuck your chin in slightly. Rather than just strolling, walk briskly to a point at which resistance occurs, where you feel like saying, 'This is difficult'.

Add some weight Before you head out on a walk, place a bundle of books in your backpack, or buy hand-held weights to increase the kilojoule-burning power of your walk.

 LITTLE TRICKS KEEP YOU MOTIVATED. For example, pick a tree and, imagining there is an elastic band extending from it to your waist and that it's pulling you forwards, walk really quickly, just till you reach it. Then drop back to your original speed.

Tame back pain

Perhaps it's the hours spent hunched over the computer keyboard, or perhaps it's the result of heaving furniture around last weekend. Whatever the cause of your back pain, there are plenty of ways to manage it and, hopefully, to prevent future flare ups.

Make your environment back friendly Sleep on a firm mattress and curl up on your side with a pillow between your knees. Choose chairs that support your lower back. Rethink activities that can bring on an attack.

Exercise regularly The only time you should avoid activity is during an acute attack. Aerobic activities such as brisk walking, and exercises such as stomach crunches that strengthen your back and stomach muscles are particularly important.

Try massage Apart from feeling wonderful, the rubbing, pushing and kneading all increase circulation to the back and relax tense muscles.

Give acupuncture a go By stimulating the flow of blood, lymph and chi – what the Chinese call life force or energy – this therapy spurs the release of endorphins, your body's natural pain-killers.

Re-educate your body Both Feldenkrais and Alexander Technique practitioners can show you stretching and postural exercises to eliminate alignment problems or muscle weaknesses, and teach you new ways to move, lift and bend without injuring yourself.

Ask a chiropractor By manipulating the joints, both chiropractic and osteopathic treatments can reduce swelling and muscle spasms.

 USE RELAXATION TECHNIQUES. Stress and anxiety cause your body to tense up, worsening and triggering back pain. Relaxation techniques will help break this cycle.

Wake up refreshed

Sleep is that golden chain that ties our health and our bodies together.

THOMAS DEKKER, DRAMATIST (1570–1632)

More than half of all women aged between 30 and 60 have trouble sleeping. Lack of sleep can do more than make you crabby, it can dull memory, reduce concentration and compromise the immune system. Think you need drugs? Think again. According to researchers at Duke University, who tested volunteers with either attitude-changing therapy, drugs or a mix of both, your mind is the most powerful sleep aid around. Here's how to make it work for you:

Change your bedroom A dark, cool room helps you fall asleep faster when you go to bed. Cut down on noise with wall-to-wall carpeting, hanging tapestries, curtains and wearing earplugs, if necessary. Eliminate symbols of activity and sources of anxiety, such as televisions, phones, computers, exercise equipment and piles of clutter.

Establish comforting bedtime habits If you pay bills just before going to bed, you won't nod off easily.

Keep sleep stress free Schedule 30 minutes of 'worry time' during the day, well before bedtime, so you don't start fretting when you hit the pillow. Make a list of the things you're anxious about, and how you're going to cope with them. Then do a Scarlett O'Hara and promise yourself you'll think about them tomorrow.

Calm your brain Protein foods contain the amino acid tryptophan, which the body converts to sleep-inducing chemicals. The best bedtime snack mixes protein, complex carbohydrates (to dispel amino acids other than tryptophan), and calcium (to help the brain use the tryptophan). Easiest of all: an oatmeal biscuit and a glass of milk.

Don't panic if you wake up If you tend to fall sound asleep then wake-up at midnight, it may help to know that, at least during that first part of the night, you're getting mostly deep sleep. If you're able to get back to sleep for even just a few hours, this second stage gives you several cycles of REM sleep, which enhances memory, learning and mood.

 DON'T KID YOURSELF that you can save time by cutting back on sleep. If you want your life to run smoothly and efficiently, get enough sleep.

I have to exercise in the morning before my brain figures out what I'm doing.

MARSHA DOBLE

Find good health care

You will make much better use of the time you spend at the doctor if you have a good, honest relationship with them. For those of us who approach modern medicine with more than the usual dose of scepticism, few decisions are as difficult as those that involve the health of ourselves and our families. For example, when Edward was about two years old, he woke up with a temperature of nearly 40 degrees and was vomiting violently. He rapidly became dehydrated, his eyes were sunken and his lips were cracked. I took him to hospital immediately for a frightening set of procedures to treat what turned out to be a very severe case of gastroenteritis: three days of intravenous antibiotics, a battery of blood tests and even a brain scan. The procedures were necessary, my doctor said (when she arrived at the hospital in her dressing gown), because in a baby Ed's age, bacterial infections could become potentially life-threatening. I decided to follow her advice, but I also negotiated to stay in hospital with Ed, to feed him myself, and to get him out of hospital as soon as possible. I also started him on a course of immune-boosting herbs and supplements with my naturopath – all of which I discussed with my doctor.

Although not all cases are as dramatic as this one, I am recounting the story because I know that each day thousands of us must make similar decisions about what's best for our health. Whatever you do, don't be rigid in your thinking – either by demanding antibiotics for every sniffle, or categorically refusing them when they're likely to help. Instead, keep an open mind about treatment options and build a relationship of trust with both your doctor and any other practitioners you wish to consider.

 GET THE BEST ADVICE. For me, the best advice is to share information with your conventional doctor – don't just listen to what they say and then go home and start using herbal remedies or anything else on your own. Tell your doctor what you're doing and what you've found to be effective, and if they're too hidebound and prejudiced, find another doctor.

Get back into those jeans

I never worry about diets. The only carrots that interest me are the number you get in a diamond.

MAE WEST

It's awfully easy to put on that extra five kilos, but it's just as easy to lose them. Small changes go a long way towards helping you reach a healthy weight, without making you feel deprived.

Jump up and down Start the day by skipping for 5 minutes.

Have some fibre first-up Breakfasting on fibre-dense multigrain toast or wholegrain cereal makes you less likely to feel empty by mid-morning.

Replace at least one sugary drink a day Instead of a soft drink, fruit juice or a sweetened coffee, choose a glass of water or green tea, which contains epigallocatechin gallate, a substance thought to curb appetite.

Avoid take away Home-cooked food is more likely to be low in fat and kilojoules.

Use less fat Rather than sloshing food in oil or butter, put extra virgin olive oil in a mist sprayer and top up with water; use to spritz the pot or frypan.

Use a smaller plate This simple trick reduces the food you can fit on your plate.

Brush your teeth The minty taste sends a message to your brain that you've eaten.

Pick fruit Whole fruit contains fewer kilojoules than fruit juice, and will leave you feeling more satisfied. Keep a bowl of bite-sized fruit, such as grapes or blueberries, on hand to nibble when you feel peckish. Peel ladyfinger bananas and freeze them (they'll stay OK for a week), then enjoy 'ice-cream' when you crave a sweet treat.

Don't just sit there Keep your arms busy while watching TV by doing biceps curls with hand-held weights.

 SWAP HANDS. Holding your fork in your non-dominant hand when eating will slow your pace and help you realise when you're full, making you more conscious of overeating.

Avoid food traps

You try to be health conscious; you choose wholegrain bread over white, and look for low-fat everything. However, many so-called healthy foods harbour excessive amounts of sugar, salt and saturated fats. Here's what to look for, and what to avoid:

Breakfast cereal This should have a short ingredients list that starts with whole grains. It should also have 5 g or more of fibre per serving. If your favourite brand is low in fibre, stir in a tablespoon or two of oat bran.

Fruit snacks Yoghurt-covered raisins and fruit leathers take perfectly good fruit and add sugar and saturated fat. Opt for unadorned fruits and vegetables instead. Dried fruit, such as apricots or raisins, is nutritious but kilojoule-dense, so make it a small snack.

Juice It satisfies thirst, not hunger, so you can consume a lot of kilojoules without realising. Juice also lacks fibre, which is important for good digestion and blood sugar control. This can be a problem for kids, who tend to be heavy juice drinkers. Buy the 100 per cent juice varieties – just limit your intake. If you're thirsty, combine a 50:50 blend of juice and sparkling water.

Soup Like other highly-processed foods, this is often packed with sodium. Cream soups are notoriously high in saturated fat and partially hydrogenated fat, which contribute to heart disease. If you don't have time to make your own, look for a vegetable soup with less then 500 mg of sodium per serve and boost the protein and fibre by stirring in a can of three bean mix.

Yoghurt Grab a yoghurt and you're getting calcium and lots of beneficial bacteria, right? Unfortunately, many yoghurts can contain up to 1 tablespoon of added sugar per cup, or they may contain the artificial sweetener aspartame. Learn to love the tangy flavour of plain low-fat yoghurt. Add your own fresh or dried fruit and a teaspoon of raw honey.

 GRAZE THROUGH THE DAY. Eating too much at one meal can make you sleepy. Breaking your food intake into several small meals rather than the traditional two or three helps maintain even energy levels.

Take out nutritional insurance

Supplements offer real benefits to help prevent major health problems, including such serious killers as heart disease, and can reduce or even eliminate the need to take drugs. They're a must in every busy woman's medicine cabinet, to ensure you're getting the nutrients you need in spite of a hectic schedule. Here are some examples:

Calcium Builds stronger bones and helps prevent osteoporosis, which can lead to crippling fractures. A study in the *New England Journal of Medicine* found that taking 1000 mg of supplemental calcium a day slowed bone loss in post-menopausal women by 43 per cent.

Evening primrose oil Contains essential fatty acids, including gamma-linolenic acid, or GLA, which benefit inflammatory conditions such as arthritis, pre-menstrual syndrome, and psoriasis.

Fish oil Reduces the risk of heart disease and eases symptoms related to some forms of arthritis and depression. It appears to prevent blood clots and, at doses of up to 6 grams per day, may also reduce levels of triglycerides – blood fats associated with an increased risk of heart disease.

Multivitamins Taking a good quality, high potency formula each day increases blood levels of nutrients believed to fight various illnesses, including cancer and heart disease.

Niacin This B vitamin lowers your risk of heart disease by reducing LDL ('bad') cholesterol while boosting HDL (the 'good' kind). However, a variety of other health conditions, including diabetes and gout, may be worsened by it, so check with your doctor first.

 GET A BLOOD TEST. Iron deficiency affects as many as 40 per cent of pre-menopausal women. Our bodies are mostly able to absorb what we need from food but among healthy women of childbearing age – especially those with heavy periods – iron stores can run low. A simple blood test can confirm whether it's a problem for you.

Age-proof your brain

The cognitive decline often associated with ageing – like memory loss and a general lack of sharpness – is not inevitable if you eat the right foods and take certain supplements. The following key nutrients help keep your brain working at its peak:

B vitamins These assist with the production of neurotransmitters like dopamine and serotonin. In addition, vitamin B12 helps produce the neurotransmitter acetylcholine, which allows nerve cells to transmit messages from your memory. Foods rich in B vitamins include dairy products, eggs, fish, lean meats, legumes and nuts.

Anti-oxidants The most important ones for memory are vitamins E and C because they fight excess free radicals that cause the oxidative damage that wears out your brain cells and keeps them from communicating with each other. Fruits and vegetables that are particularly high in vitamin E include almonds, avocadoes and sunflower seeds; vitamin C-rich foods include broccoli, kiwifruit and red capsicums.

Magnesium, iron and zinc These are said to maintain brain health: magnesium stabilises brainwave patterns and increases blood flow to the brain; iron and zinc both play significant roles in your ability to concentrate, especially on demanding tasks that involve memory and reasoning. You can get magnesium by eating foods like artichokes, avocados, legumes, nuts and whole grains. Iron and zinc tend to be found in the same foods, and good sources for both include lean red meat, legumes (including soybean products like tofu and tempeh), poultry and whole grains.

Omega-3 fats A diet rich in omega-3 fats helps keep the lining of your brain cells flexible so that memory messages can pass easily between them. You should eat foods rich in omega-3 fats every day. Good sources include cold-water fish such as salmon; sardines, tuna and trout; flaxseed oil; and eggs.

 CHECK YOUR MEDICATION. Some medications, such as diuretics, interfere with the absorption of nutrients, especially potassium and magnesium. If you're concerned, ask your doctor.

What if they snore?

Dear, never forget one small point. It's my business.
You just work here.

ELIZABETH ARDEN, IN A NOTE TO HER HUSBAND

How can you get a good night's sleep when the problem is lying right next to you? Sleep deprivation doesn't just ruin your mood, health and looks, it can also force one partner to move out of the bed altogether and into another room, which can have serious repercussions for the relationship. Here are some ideas:

Try different options Think about earplugs, for a start, or twin mattresses pushed together, or dual control electric blankets. A stubborn problem merits a trip to a sleep disorders clinic specialising in the diagnosis and treatment of conditions such as sleep apnoea and restless legs syndrome.

Get back to sleep If you're the woken-uppee as opposed to the waker-upper, you need to find a technique for winding back down again. For example, learn to consciously relax one muscle group at a time, rather than staying awake.

Don't ignore the problem It's unlikely to go away of its own accord, and things can get nasty when two people have trouble sleeping together. Communicate your feelings as reasonably as you can, with the ultimate goal of a compromise.

 DON'T FORGO CUDDLES. Too many mornings waking up alone can dilute closeness and feed resentment. When sleeping apart is the only way to get some rest, don't let sex fall by the wayside. If you're too tired in the evening, make a date for Sunday morning!

Keep it simple

Food is an important part of a balanced diet.

FRAN LEBOWITZ, WRITER AND HUMORIST

The good news is that once you look past the experts and the breakthroughs (and the food companies who are sponsoring the research!), what we should actually be eating is remarkably straightforward. Stick with these principles:

Swap bad fats for good fats Aim to eat less saturated fat (the kind abundant in fatty cuts of meat and full-fat dairy products) and trans fats (the hydrogenated kinds in margarine and commercial baked goods). Brush bread with olive oil or mashed avocado instead of butter, and cook with olive or canola oil; all are rich in mono-unsaturated fats which reduce your risk of cardiovascular disease.

Eat more vegetables Eat Asian-style and regard meat, poultry or fish as a savoury accent to your meal – not the main part. Try to have one vegetarian day a week.

Eat fish twice a week Salmon and other fatty fish are richest in the heart-healthy omega-3 fatty acids, but canned or fresh tuna is also good – and it's cheaper.

Put leafy greens on every plate They are abundant in omega-3 fatty acids and B vitamins, including folic acid, and fibre.

Go for whole grains Trade white flour products for dark varieties made with whole-wheat flour. Diets rich in whole grains have been shown to lower the risk of heart disease, diabetes, cancer and intestinal troubles like diverticulitis.

Got a sweet tooth? Satisfy it with the most delicious fruit you can find. Apart from being high in fibre, fruit is also a great source of anti-oxidants such as vitamin C, which may protect against cancer, heart disease and age-related ailments including macular degeneration.

Kick the white habit White rice and potatoes make blood sugar surge. You don't have to spurn all starches – for example, brown rice and less starchy small red potatoes are better because they're digested slowly – but think of them as a treat, not a staple.

 USE FLAVOUR BOOSTERS to make food come alive. Worcestershire sauce, soy sauce, fresh, grated ginger, or aromatic cumin, tarragon and lashings of black pepper can all enhance otherwise bland foods.

No woman can be handsome by the force of her features alone, any more than she can be witty by only the help of speech.

LANGSTON HUGHES

Feel good in your skin

A woman's body is a work of art. A man's body is utilitarian.
It's for getting around. It's like a Jeep.

ELAINE, *SEINFELD* (ON WHY MEN SHOULDN'T WALK AROUND NAKED)

Do you like your body? Most women can't answer 'yes' to this question. Midlife brings a variety of physical changes that can revive old insecurities. Crow's feet, love handles and tuckshop arms keep us from going swimming, making love or dancing – the very things that make us feel good about ourselves! It's far better to be happy in the body you're in, than to pine for lost youthful looks. And the key to getting comfortable with your shape is to learn to see your body in a new way:

Write down five things you like about your body Now go and stand in front of a full-length mirror. Shut your eyes, and think about why you like one of the things on your list – your hands, perhaps –and say the reasons out loud: 'I like the way my nails are smooth and oval; my hands are graceful yet strong; I like wearing rings to show them off, and people often compliment me on them.' Open your eyes and look straight at your hands in the mirror, turning them this way and that. Repeat the exercise, visualising the next thing on your list.

Write down five things you don't like Repeat the mirror-viewing exercise with one difference: use neutral descriptions for the different body features, rather than emotive or judgemental ones. For example, instead of, 'I hate my thighs, they're huge and flabby', say, 'My thighs are very curvy and feminine, which means I look much better in a skirt than in tight pants'. If you're really distressed by one or more of the disliked things, just work through a couple and save the rest for another session.

Feel good naked Repeat the entire exercise, thinking and talking about both the positives and the negatives – but this time, do it without your clothes on. The aim of the exercise is to reprogram yourself to be able to look at your body without feeling bad.

 OPEN YOUR EYES to the women around you. Every time I go to the local pool, I'm reminded that beauty comes in a remarkable variety of shapes and sizes.

Stay safe

If that little voice inside you tells you that something or someone spells danger to you and your family, take action immediately. Having your bag or wallet stolen or your house burgled is one of the most infuriating and time-consuming things that can happen to you. To stay in control and safe wherever you are, remember:

Don't put your keys in plant pots or mailboxes They are the first places that a burglar will look. Never put your name and address on keys.

Don't open the door without seeing who it is Always ask for identification from service people, even if you are expecting them.

Never give address or credit card details to market research companies Don't answer questions that ask how many people live in your household, or what they do for a living.

Be alert when out Notice your surroundings – who is in front of you and behind you. If you think you are being followed, walk immediately towards an area with other people and good lighting. If you're driving and think you're being followed, or someone gestures that there's something wrong with your car, don't drive home or pull over; note the number plate and drive straightaway to a police station or any open business and report the incident.

Carry a shrill whistle in your bag and walk with confidence Thieves and pickpockets invariably speak of picking a target who 'looked like a victim'.

Hold your bag close to your body You should preferably have the strap diagonally across your chest. Handle your money and credit cards carefully – don't display them unnecessarily.

Don't sit near doors or exits on buses, trams or trains Statistics show that you are more vulnerable to being attacked or pulled off the vehicle in those spots.

Be cautious in lifts Always check who else is in there and stand near the controls; if you are attacked, hit the alarm.

Drive safely Check the back seats and floor of your car before getting in. Lock car doors and put the windows up. Never put your handbag on the passenger seat – it may tempt a thief to smash the window and grab it. Put it on the floor instead.

 DON'T MAKE YOURSELF A TARGET. Don't carry large shopping bags unless you are going straight to your car – heavy loads only slow you down and make you clumsy.

Quick fixes

Diet, exercise, sleep and other long-term habits are the foundations of looking good. But sometimes you need a quickfix to look better straightaway. Try these tricks:

Move gracefully If you don't, you look old and tired. Poor posture can result from even just slinging your handbag or briefcase over the same shoulder every day.

Try do-it-yourself reflexology If you're relaxed, you look better. Stimulating the pressure points on your feet reduces stress. Press your thumb into your solar plexus point, located just below the ball of your foot. Hold and repeat on your other foot.

Mist your face Dull, dry skin magnifies fine lines, so spritz on this recipe whenever skin feels tight: combine 1 cup of still mineral water, $^1/_2$ cup of witch-hazel, and 3 drops of chamomile oil in a spray bottle. Stored in a cool dry place, it keeps indefinitely.

Heal rough hands Before bedtime, slather your hands with almond or apricot kernel oil. Slip on cotton gloves (or socks), and sleep with them on. By morning your hands will be baby soft and smooth.

Banish the bloat Retaining water can make you look and feel heavier. Diuretic herbs such as horsetail (*Equisetum arvense*) or dandelion (*Taraxacum officinale*) can help. Don't exceed recommended dosages because you can lose essential minerals.

Try a course of Siberian ginseng (*Eleutherococcus senticosus*) The energy you feel is sustained over time, rather than a quick jolt, like a caffeine hit.

Think loving thoughts Sit quietly by yourself for 15 minutes with your eyes closed. Gently bring to mind a happy memory of a friend, a parent or a child. Breathe in deeply through your nose for four counts – then exhale through your mouth for eight counts. Happy, positive thoughts make you glow from the inside out.

 USE THE MAKE-UP ARTIST'S SECRET WEAPON – a cold teaspoon. Place two in the freezer for a few minutes, then hold over puffy eyes. The spoons' bowls fit the contours of the eye perfectly and, unlike cucumber slices, the metal stays cold long enough to do the trick.

Fake good looks

Youth is something very new: twenty years ago, no one mentioned it.

COCO CHANEL

Do you think the only way to look ten years younger is to go under the knife? No way. Smart cosmetic choices and easy tricks of the beauty trade do the job for a lot less money and pain.

Smooth forehead wrinkles The new light-reflecting foundations and powders literally scatter light over the surface of your skin, blurring flaws and evening out skin tone, giving your skin a healthy sheen. After cleansing and moisturising your face, smooth on one of these all-in-one optical-illusion foundations. To further downplay wrinkles, dot along them with a light-reflecting pencil, blend the edges, then dust with translucent powder.

Lift droopy eyes Gently tweeze your brows. If you show more of the brow bone it gives the illusion of lifted lids. Use a neutral-coloured eye shadow – a bone or pale pink – rather than a dark colour, which can make your eyes look heavy.

Get rid of dark under-eye circles Some people are born with a propensity towards dark circles; others develop them as the skin in this area begins to thin, which allows colour from blood vessels to show through. Look for an opaque concealer that's a shade lighter than your foundation. Blend with your ring finger, then set with a thin layer of translucent powder.

Erase lip lines Keep your lipstick from accentuating those fine lines around your mouth. Exfoliate your lips by massaging them briskly with a warm face washer, then moisturise as usual. Dab foundation onto the lines around your lips and blend with a sponge. Then use a tissue lightly dusted with loose powder to blot the area and prevent the colour from feathering. Remember that dark-coloured lipstick will make your lips look narrower.

 LOOK MORE ALERT. Using a lash curler can make you look more alert. Heat it with a hairdryer for a few seconds to make it even more effective.

Planning essentials
The health checks

After 40, most women begin to find out what it means to 'feel your age'. The little signs – finding it harder to keep the extra weight off, or tiring more easily – aren't serious, but they should remind you not to take your health for granted. Consider scheduling some or all of the following tests:

Blood pressure Test at least once a year. Checks can be part of any appointment.

Bone density test Most doctors recommend having this done at 50, but if you are in a high-risk category (if you are Asian or Caucasian, small-boned, have a low calcium intake, a family history of osteoporosis and/or a history of heavy drinking or smoking) it may be prudent to have it done earlier.

Breast health Discuss the pros and cons of regular mammograms with your doctor – opinions vary. Also ask your doctor to examine your breasts as part of your regular check-ups, and get into the habit of examining yourself at least once a month.

Cholesterol test Test every three years or more often, according to doctor's advice.

Colorectal cancer screenings Different doctors may suggest different time spans for this twin test of a colonoscopy with a barium enema, and a digital rectal examination, depending on family history.

Dental A check-up and professional clean once every six months is ideal.

Faecal occult blood test This can be an early warning sign of colon cancer or other gastrointestinal problems.

Fasting plasma glucose test This is imperative for anyone with a history of diabetes, especially if they're overweight.

Pelvic examination and PAP test This should be done once a year. Over half of all cervical cancers are diagnosed in women between the ages of 50 and 70.

Skin cancer Check thoroughly in front of a mirror at least once a month; in addition, ask your doctor to check for early skin cancers, or visit the Skin Cancer Council.

Vision Test every two years after 40, or more often if you have diabetes or a family history of macular degeneration or glaucoma.

The shopping list

As a mother of sons, I know first-hand what a relentless task it is to keep the cupboards stocked with food. It seems no matter what I buy, or how much, it's never enough. The fridge door thumps to-and-fro like a friendly labrador's tail, and if they have friends over to visit, they'll eat everything that isn't nailed down or with a skull and crossbones. You can at least make the job easier by sticking to a list so you always have the right ingredients in your pantry, fridge and freezer. It also helps you stay within a budget, by reducing the tendency to impulse-buy. Here's how:

Make a master list On your computer, create a list of all the major ingredients and grocery staples you use in your everyday cooking. Start with the pantry: olive oil, mustard, soy sauce, canned beans, canned tomatoes, pasta, rice, bread, canned tuna and salmon. Now, move on to the fridge: eggs, butter or margarine, yoghurt, cheese. List the fruit and vegetables you like to have on hand. If you have a freezer, add bread or bread rolls, meat and sausages, frozen vegetables, pizza bases. Print the list out every week and see what you've run out of, highlighting what you need before going shopping.

Identify favourite dinners There is bound to be a selection of anywhere between five and ten basic meals that you and your family eat on a regular basis – perhaps it's roast chicken, or a cheesy pasta bake, or perhaps you barbecue regularly. List the ingredients that you need for these reliable recipes, ensure they're on your master list, and you'll always have the makings of an easy and delicious dinner that will please everyone.

Keep a running list The family noticeboard is a handy place to add reminders for other items that run out in the meantime.

Plan ahead Where possible, plan a week's worth of menus ahead of time. You can even try for two weeks, to cut down trips to the supermarket. You may not cook exactly what you'd planned to on the day you'd planned it, but you'll have a pretty good idea of what you'll be doing – and spending – for the next fortnight. And buy non-perishables in bulk if you can. It saves you time and can save you money.

I think you have to take charge of your own life and understand that you're either going to live somebody else's dream, or live your own dream.

WILMA MANKILLER, FIRST WOMAN CHIEF, CHEROKEE NATION

Work systems that work

When home is your office

The huge variety of demands on a woman's time can often make it necessary for her to figure out alternatives to a standard nine-to-five job. Many work styles and careers are better suited to an out-of-office arrangement, and often employers find it an advantage, for example, when downsizing a work force or reducing expenses or office space.

Options include working part-time, working from home, flexitime and job-share arrangements, and working as a temp. The big advantage of these options is that they give women a choice about when and how to work. You can establish a balance between work and family life, and stay on track with your career. Plus you waste less time travelling; you save money on fares, lunches and clothes; you can schedule work according to your unique body clock, whether you're a morning person or a night owl; you can claim at least some tax-deductible business expenses; and, if you're a mum, you can usually be there when your kids come home. So, is it for you? Work through these points first:

Costs and benefits Some companies will continue to pay health benefits and superannuation to part-time employees, others won't. Some of your set-up costs might be offset by worthwhile tax deductions. Look into the options with your accountant.

Money versus time You need to weigh up initial financial disadvantage against the benefits of having more time and flexibility.

Both sides should be clear about the arrangement If part-time work or job-sharing is your choice then be specific about your goals: let your employer know what you're capable of doing, what you hope to achieve, and how it will benefit them. Have a contract or letter of agreement drawn up.

Stay in touch If you are planning to telecommute, make sure you install a separate phone line for business, schedule weekly teleconferences with your boss and colleagues, and equip yourself with reliable computer hardware and a fast Internet Service Provider.

MAKE SURE PEOPLE CAN REACH YOU. Provide several ways for co-workers and clients to reach you if it's urgent – phone, email, pager, mobile phone.

The five kid commandments

Nothing brings you back to earth more than coming home from parliament to two kids for whom the most important issue of the day is whether they can go to the dance that night.

JANINE HAINES, AUSTRALIAN POLITICIAN

If your work and your kids are under the same roof, these are the non-negotiables that will help you manage:

1. Don't let them interrupt when you're on the phone When my kids were small and I was working, I taught them that I was only to be disturbed 'if there was blood'. Make them write what they want on a piece of paper and put it in front of you, then you can decide whether it can wait, or whether you will cut the call short.

2. Schedule important meetings and calls for kids' down time If they're small, this could be while they're having a nap; if they're older, while they're doing homework.

3. Plan ahead for the school holidays Investigate holiday care programs, local community courses, sports clinics, and camps. Set up a list of possible backups for childcare. Try to be more flexible than usual about your schedule. For example, trade off an early morning excursion to the pool or beach with your kids, for a quiet afternoon so you can do some catching up.

4. Get to know your local public library It's amazing how much time, money and running around you can save yourself. Need advice about council-run craft programs, books for a school project or a directory of kids' clubs? First stop: the library.

5. Let them help Even littlies are quite capable of folding letters, stuffing envelopes, sticking on labels and perhaps sorting and binning old magazines and files. And it can be fun.

 SET BOUNDARIES. Children need to know when you are working and when you are 'at home'.

Stay motivated

Problems arise when working from home if you find it hard to get started and stay motivated without others' input. Here's how to overcome the main traps:

Create a clear physical line between your workplace and the rest of your home Partitioning or curtaining your workplace off sends a clear signal that it is not family space and can help you get your work done. So does staying away from high-traffic, high-noise areas, like the kitchen.

Focus on your 'real' work Don't get distracted with hanging out a load of washing, or going to the shops first. By all means, get essential chores done before your start-up time – but not after. If you do, it means that you're not taking your real work seriously, that you see the chores as more important.

Process quick administrative jobs first For example, reply to emails, or fill out time sheets, before moving on to the main task for the day.

Be clear on when you'll be available Friends and family, in particular, think that if you're at home you're not really working, and therefore you won't mind being interrupted.

Break tasks up This is an absolute must if you're a new mum working from home, because you will only have little chunks of time between baby's nap and feed times.

Set a time frame for each job And stick to it.

Know your limits Recognise and respect the signals that mean you're tired, and that it's time to stop.

 KICK-START YOUR DAY by establishing a small, pleasant habit that puts you in the right frame of mind. This could be as simple as quickly scanning the newspaper, or doing 15 minutes of stretching.

Smart space management

Stand up to your obstacles and do something about them. You will find that they haven't half the strength you think they have.

NORMAN VINCENT PEALE, MINISTER

When setting up your work space, keep these two questions in mind: what information and tools must you be able to access easily? And how will you be able to find items that you've put away? Let's start with the three Rs – Reduce, Refer, Rearrange.

Reduce by throwing out as much as possible Touch every binder, book, file, box and newspaper. Look first at recycling as much of the excess paper as you can.

Refer information and backup documents For projects that you are no longer involved with, you can refer them to the person who is working on them. If there is no one to refer the item to, but it does retain historical value, e.g. backup computer disks, then box and label them and move them out of your work space. They should be stored somewhere safe, but not take up critical space where you work.

Rearrange the remaining items The guiding principle, when sorting, is to put like things together. Group together all reference manuals, for example, course materials or books by subject. Gather together loose papers. Put those that belong in your filing system in a stack to be filed. Hole-punch the rest (things such as call sheets and minutes of meetings) and logically order them in binders.

 CLEAR YOUR WORK SPACE. Move or bin general household items that have encroached on your work space – empty food containers, newspapers and other junk.

Organise your work flow

There's no right or wrong way to manage your work flow – what works for you is what's right. However, there's a quick, 2-minute test to see whether your system is working: if you can't find a document or item that you're looking for in under 2 minutes, it's time to reorganise. These tips will put you in control:

Keep your work space clear Reserve it for items you use regularly, e.g. your in/out tray, computer, disk box, calendar, message pad. Supplies you only reach for occasionally (manila folders, stapler, staples, paper, labels, etc.) should be kept in a drawer or cupboard. Shelve reference materials (e.g. dictionary, reports, books).

Only have what you're working on right now in front of you Don't have lots of different projects spread out over your work surface. Don't leave letters, memos or reports lying on top of your desk.

Check your filing- and in-trays Spend, say, 20 minutes a day on clearing them. A little organising each day means you will reach the bottom of the stack. Clear out finished jobs at least once a day, and either distribute them, or file them.

Don't clutter noticeboards Regularly remove information that is no longer relevant. Ask yourself: do I need this? Why? What happens to it next?

Rationalise your stationery Do you really need three pairs of scissors, Post-it notes in every size, and dozens of paper clips littering the bottom of the drawers?

Put your phone on the right side (for you) of the desk The same goes for fresh pencils, pens and notepads. Every single one of us has wasted time looking for a pen that works or a pencil that's not broken, just to write down a phone message.

Put things away when you've finished with them If you do it as you go, you'll save time by not having to clean up a big mess.

 ARRANGE YOUR DESK. The more you use something, the closer it should be to you. Frequency of use is the key to arranging your desk.

Tame the paper tiger

Are you drowning in a sea of paper? There's nothing more disheartening and overwhelming than a huge stack of incoming paperwork. It's hard to get rid of too – there's something about the importance of the printed word on paper that causes even the most conscientious among us to put off throwing it out. However, the worst thing you can do is to scan an item and then put it back, thinking you'll come back to it another time. Here's how to win the paper war:

Sort, categorise and discard papers and opened mail immediately You should preferably do this at the same time each day. Quickly glance over every piece of mail and every memo or email message you have received. If it looks as if it's potentially important, file it right away in a folder marked 'pending', or delegate it to someone else to take care of. If it's not relevant or it's something you'll never look at again, trash it. Handle your home mail the same way.

Be informal A short handwritten reply or an email is quicker than a memo or letter. There are bound to be important incoming letters you need to keep but, generally speaking, when you've answered a card or a letter, you should toss it. The same goes for Christmas cards. Update your own address book as necessary, and then recycle the cards.

Be ruthless Throw out catalogues, unnecessary newsletters, circulars and the like, straightaway.

✳ FOLLOW THE THREE Ds: either Do it straightaway, Delegate and pass it on to someone else, or Ditch it.

File it and find it

If you hate filing, you're not alone. It's not just that it's a boring, repetitive task – it's the agony of deciding whether to keep a piece of paper or throw it away, and the teeth-gnashing effect of forgetting where something's filed. Creating well-organised files makes the task bearable. Here's how:

Buy a good quality suspension filing cabinet Position it so that it is convenient and accessible. Keeping receipts and documents in shoeboxes is a one-way ticket to chaos.

Set aside enough time If you are establishing files (or significantly overhauling them), block out at least an afternoon.

Decide on a system For my money, alphabetical listing works best. File related documents under the letter of the 'umbrella' subject, e.g. file all warranties, registration and insurance documents under C for Car. The test of your system is to be able to retrieve something again, so give files names that have an immediate association for you.

Head files with a noun For example, Archives, Bills, Cheque Accounts, Instruction Manuals, Savings Accounts, School Papers and Tax. Miscellaneous or Other are catch-all traps. Avoid labelling files with a date or adjective.

File chronologically When adding documents, place the most recent at the front.

Store large or bulky items on shelves Things like reports, books and magazines can be kept on shelves or in archive boxes, not in your filing cabinet.

Use pop-up plastic folder tabs Use your best printing and a sharp, fine-tipped pen (pencils smudge). Write your labels in upper and lower case. This is easier to read than all capitals.

Keep files lean Regularly purge them of instructions and warranties for products you no longer own, out-of-date brochures and old business cards. Research shows that 80 per cent of papers filed will never be looked at again. Ask yourself, 'If I couldn't find this paper again, could I get the information somewhere else?' If so, cull it. If you're still not sure, file it in an archive box.

 FILE IN YOUR NON-PEAK ENERGY TIME. You'll also be more alert and file more quickly if you stand up while you're doing it.

After years of banging heads against the glass ceiling, huge numbers of women of a certain age and self-awareness who are weary of adapting to environments in which they don't fit in are leaving to create companies that fit them.

JOLINE GODFREY, AUTHOR

Keep up with information

Everybody gets so much information all day long that they lose their common sense.

GERTRUDE STEIN, AUTHOR

Magazines, professional journals, newsletters, catalogues: it is easy to become overwhelmed unless you evaluate the publications you receive. Ask, 'What would happen if I didn't get this?' or, 'How often does it offer something I actually use?' Then use these tips to read more efficiently:

Read with a pen in your hand Highlight passages in reports, proposals and documents as you go along. You can also write any thoughts, comments or questions that you may have in the margins.

Don't let newspapers pile up Scan your daily paper very quickly – news summaries, usually on the outside back cover, are a great time saver. If you find an article that's important, rip out the page and put it in a file to read in the evening in front of the television, while waiting for appointments or while travelling on public transport. Then recycle the newspaper. With weekend newspapers, break them down as soon as they arrive and discard sections of no interest to you, e.g. if you're not in the market for a car or a new job, toss these sections away immediately.

Skim the table of contents in magazines If you see an article that looks interesting, rip out the pages, note the source and date if necessary, and throw the rest of the magazine or newsletter away. Once you've read the article, toss it, pass it to someone else or file it in one of the permanent files you allow yourself for reference (e.g. Cats, Diet, Garden, etc.).

Set aside 30 minutes, twice a week, for reading Schedule it in your diary.

Have newspapers and magazines delivered Not having to stop off at the newsagent or to leave the house on weekends to pick them up will save you time.

 TAKE A SPEED READING COURSE or buy a book that teaches you how to read faster. This applies especially if you read everything at the same pace.

Get rid of junk mail

If unsolicited mail – print or electronic – is becoming a time-consuming problem, here's what to do:

Get off mailing lists Advise mailing houses and direct advertisers that you wish to be taken off their lists. You can either write to them to request your name be taken off their list, or simply add a handwritten message to the bottom of the business or household mail which has come to you and return it. Senders of unsolicited mail are usually happy to cooperate if you don't want to receive their messages: most mail-outs are quite expensive, and the sender is no more interested in poorly targeted mail that won't deliver a sales result than you are in receiving it.

Complain If you still have a problem, contact the office of the Australian Direct Marketing Association in your state and ask for your name to be eliminated from all national advertising catalogue lists.

Use a 'no junk mail' sign Posting a notice on your mailbox says loud and clear that you do not wish to receive any unsolicited mail.

 NIX SPAM. If you receive unsolicited electronic mail, check the bottom of the material for the 'autoresponder' or 'unsubscribe' address. Send an email to the address with the word 'remove' in the subject heading.

Standardise letters

Remember: 'Impossible' means 'I'm possible'.

SARK, ARTIST AND POET

With both household and work-related correspondence, there are many examples of standard letters you have to send out, time and again: thankyou letters, apologies, complaints, congratulations, requests for information, invitations, and so on. You can save a lot of time by setting up standardised letters and using them over and over again for different correspondents. Just change the date, greeting, address, etc. They're especially useful for writing to your kids' teachers, asking for information for school projects; sending out work-related applications; appeals for fundraisers; and 'thanks-but-no-thanks' letters. Ready-made software packages can make you speedier and more efficient in certain tasks, such as creating databases for mailings for every conceivable occasion. Same goes for family-style software packages that contain home entertainment and educational systems.

 SEND PERSONAL NEWSLETTERS. They aren't everyone's cup of tea, but they do save time, prevent writer's cramp, and allow you to stay in touch with lots of family and friends.

Your computer

We used to have lots of questions to which there were no answers. Now, with computers, there are lots of answers to which we haven't thought up the questions.

PETER USTINOV, BRITISH ACTOR

Equip your computer system with as many productivity-boosting and timesaving tools as possible:

Do your homework Computer magazines are invaluable when you need to research the comparisons between different models.

Buy a super fast model Add lots of memory or RAM (random access memory) – at least double the minimum amount needed to run the latest software. A high-speed modem, Internet connection, a huge hard drive, printer, keyboard, mouse or trackball, and a big monitor are also needed. If you're going to be using a CD-ROM, you probably need a sound card and speakers. Depending on the nature of your work, a scanner or digital camera may also be required. Protecting yourself with an automatic backup tape drive (like a Zip) is also a good idea.

Backup, backup, backup Any data you create on your computer is vulnerable to disasters – from power surges and viruses to plain old human error. Backup everything onto diskettes, and activate the automatic 'save' function on your computer, so that it saves your work every 15 minutes.

Buy a good surge protector You should do this especially if you live in an area with frequent power surges.

Keep all of your computer's documents Including any manuals, warranties and software installation CDs.

 ASK AN EXPERT. To increase your confidence – and to save time trying to do it yourself – hire an expert for an hour to tell you what you could be doing, and make any adjustments to hardware or install better software accordingly. Your computer dealer will be able to recommend someone. The money invested could be a tax deduction, as well as being the key to a better computer experience.

Your hard drive

A hard drive is like an electronic filing cabinet: no matter how big it is, if you keep adding files and programs without deleting anything, it will eventually become stuffed beyond its capacity. Until you actually start getting rid of old computer files and unused programs, you won't realise how much space – and time – you're wasting.

Create an archive If you're not sure whether or not you should keep a specific file, create an archive directory where you can at least get them out of the way. This is especially relevant if you're using a computer that belonged to someone before you. Chances are the person's files are still on the hard drive. Check the dates and view them, one by one.

Copy files onto floppies If you want to keep specific files, copy them onto a floppy disk and keep it in a safe place. When you save files onto a floppy, be sure to write a label for the floppy disk that describes what's on there.

Delete old programs Do you still have the DOS version of a program even though you've been using the Windows version for years? And what about the software package that you downloaded from the Internet and used for a few days, then decided that you didn't like it? Get rid of them.

✳ THROW AWAY PRINT-OUTS. Ask yourself whether you need to keep both the hard copy and the computer file. Keeping both is often pointless.

Virus protection

Some computer viruses are relatively harmless, simply introducing silly pop-up images or messages. However, many are deadly, can ruin your computer and wipe your hard drive. Be vigilant about protecting your computer from viruses:

Install and use a high quality antivirus software system The most popular are Norton and Virex, but this area changes constantly – seek advice from your computer professional. Make sure whichever software you choose is set to scan your hard drive every time you boot up, and use the virus-spotting portion of the program at all times.

Always scan floppy disks and CDs Never boot your computer with a floppy disk or CD that you haven't scanned first. Don't open attachments from people or addresses you don't recognise. Trash offers that sound too good to be true, especially if they come from a strange address. This may sound like commonsense, but people who spread computer viruses are sneaky and enjoy disguising them, which is why most of us fall victim to them through curiosity.

Update every day Up to ten new computer viruses are discovered every day, and the frequency is increasing. Most virus detection software packages require you to update regularly. You can usually make the updates for free via their websites.

Keep it clean If you do get a virus, don't panic. Go into your virus software and run the program to identify and quarantine it, or remove it. If there's still a problem, contact your computer professional. Remember that most data can still be recovered from the hard drive eventually.

 LOOK OUT FOR HOAXES. Almost as irritating as viruses are hoax emails that supposedly announce a new virus and then instruct you on how to remove it (usually by deleting some part of your basic software). If in doubt, go to a virus-tracking website like Symantec, which posts daily updates on real viruses, and also identifies hoaxes.

Planning essentials
The desk

When setting up your workplace, keep these points in mind:

Desk size and shape How large do you really need your desk to be? How much drawer space will you need?

The right chair It should have an adjustable seat, backrest and arms; a slightly forward-sloping seat cushion, so it doesn't dig into the backs of your legs; and mobility – being able to swivel, tilt, and roll on casters will give you ease of motion.

Position yourself correctly Type with a flat wrist, held at or just below elbow level, so that your forearms are at a 90-degree angle to your upper arms. Typing with a cocked wrist, either upward or downward, places extra stress on tendons and nerves. If the height of the keyboard is adjustable, it's easy to achieve this 90-degree position. If the keyboard is sitting on a desk or table whose height cannot be changed, raise your chair to the proper height and use a footrest to support your feet. Never rest your wrists on the edge of the work surface as this puts additional pressure on those same tendons and nerves. Use a padded wrist rest or palm rest.

Angle your monitor You should be able to look straight at the screen without tilting your head up or down. Adjust the settings to reduce screen glare. Consider installing an anti-glare screen. To minimise the strain on your neck, attach a copy holder to the side of your monitor. This holds papers right next to the screen, minimising eye and neck movement.

Get a footrest An important and often overlooked item, it can reduce the pressure on the backs of your thighs, minimise lower back pain and improve the circulation of blood throughout your body.

Don't work in bad light Ideally, you want light bright enough for you to easily read your papers, while at the same time providing enough indirect light so that you can work at your computer without seeing glare. You may need to install adjustable blinds on windows.

The equipment

In addition to your desk and basics such as calculator, clock, address book or card holders for contacts, desk lamp, diary, noticeboard, paper trays and rubbish bin, you will need:

A phone Choose a model with features that enhance productivity, e.g. push-button dialling; an LED display to identify the source of incoming calls; memory dial; conference calling, so you can link multiple parties to the same call; a redial button; a message indicator and call waiting indicator; and voicemail. If you spend a lot of time on the telephone, try a telephone headset instead of the traditional handset.

A mobile phone Before you get the newest high-tech model and sign up for a payment plan, consider your calling patterns. If you're one of the 80 per cent of people who rarely uses your phone outside your calling area, a local plan makes more sense. Choose a plan where the airtime charges are least during your busiest periods.

A fax machine Avoid machines that use thermal paper because it is difficult to handle and faxes printed on it fade over time. Investigate options that let you fax directly from your computer thereby eliminating the need for paper.

A scanner This saves time by transforming hard copy material into editable files that you can incorporate directly into your document without re-keying.

A photocopier You can get small home models for less than $600. If your business does not yet justify such an investment, check out mail service and/or printing companies that provide photocopying services (via a smart card for self-service operation at a much cheaper rate than a pharmacy or newsagent, and with faster machines).

Inspiration Have the things you love around you and it will be a pleasure to be in your office – photos of friends and family, a posy of flowers, and colourful pictures will all support your quest for success.

Don't cook. Don't clean. No man will ever make love to a woman because she waxed the linoleum – 'My God, the floor's immaculate. Lie down, you hot bitch'.

JOAN RIVERS, TALK SHOW HOST

Make your house work

Recycle it

Just about every inanimate object can be reused by someone else. Local councils have programs to take away paper, plastic, glass and garden refuse, as well as providing regular clean-up initiatives that save you from going to the tip. Government departments offer brochures or web-accessible advice on where to find and buy recycled materials, including timber, office supplies and paper, garden furniture, packaging and car accessories. Many charities are happy to collect clothing, rags and furniture, which may then be sold or recycled at thrift shops.

Clothes If you no longer wear or fit into something, give it to someone who needs it or recycle it into something else. Don't forget old woollens, raincoats and shoes that aren't so obvious when you open the wardrobe door, or which might be stored elsewhere. Recycled children's clothing shops take good quality baby items, including nappies, toys and furniture, on consignment. You should keep a selection of old pantyhose, shoes, T-shirts, leotards, tea towels, hats and bags ready for school concert costumes. My boys have been pirates, two wise men, ghosts, spacemen and, on one memorable occasion, an adorable elf (though Edward says I'm a dead woman if I show anyone the photos).

Books Sell them to a second-hand bookstore or give them to a school library. Pass on those special books that you have loved but won't read again to friends or family.

Magazines Give them to a school, a hospital, a retirement village or nursing home full of people who will be glad of them. Same goes for your local hairdressing salon, local medical practice or dental surgery; or, give them to the local kindergarten for children to cut up.

 MAKE MONEY. Get together with a group of friends and organise a market stall or giant garage sale to sell things you don't want anymore. You will make money and have fun.

Put it away

There are three ways to get things done: do it yourself, employ someone, or forbid your children to do it.

MONTA CRANE, AUTHOR

My mother always used to say, 'A place for everything, and everything in its place'. A lot of the junk that's messing up your house is probably just stuff that should be somewhere else. Of course, putting things in their place isn't that easy if you're fresh out of places. Here are some ideas:

Everything has to justify being there Walk through each room and quickly assess each item displayed. Ask yourself why you are keeping it. If it has a function, does it work? Do you enjoy seeing it? Be critical. Remove anything that fails the test and either discard it, sell it, or give it away.

Never leave a room empty-handed If you brought something into a room, take it out with you the next time you leave. Take things upstairs if you are going there, e.g. put folded washing on the step ready for when you next go upstairs. Take everything out of the car that was added on the last trip. Train your family or flatmates to take their stuff with them as they go too.

Fix it when it happens Pick up things when they drop, wipe up spills when they happen, and wash dishes and wipe down benchtops before the food dries and goes hard. The good news is that this will actually save you time – it will take a lot longer to wipe up a dried-up spill than a fresh one. The bad news is that it's not going to work unless you have the cooperation of everyone else in the household. Call a family meeting and get everyone to agree to the, 'Place for everything, and everything in its place', rule. Agree on rewards for adhering to the terms – and punishments for infringing them.

✳ DON'T WASTE TIME. If you spend 10 minutes a day looking for things that aren't in the right place, you waste more than 60 hours a year!

Cut down on housework

I don't like sitting on a sofa that's covered with clothes and books, or tripping over toys or newspapers as I move around a room – but I also resent giving up time on housework that I'd rather spend on other things. These tips will help:

Ask, 'What's more important?' Faced with a choice between folding the washing or taking your child for a walk around the block – go for the walk.

Close doors Do only what is immediately necessary. Decide which rooms and areas in the home are in view or in constant use, and focus your energy on them.

Aim for low maintenance Decide which tasks are essential to do every day – for me, it's washing the dishes and taking the garbage out – and which are non-essential.

Be selective about furniture and decorations Only keeping items that are genuinely useful and/or that you really love means less stuff to clean.

Utilise wall space Identify wall space which could be utilised for book shelving or storage. Building lidded window seats are another easy storage solution.

Put ornaments away You should especially do this if you've got little children. It only makes for more dusting, not to mention the anxiety whenever anyone runs through the house.

Unclutter your lounge room Put your TV and sound system in a purpose-built cabinet or storage unit so they are out of sight when not in use. This will create an uncluttered feeling.

Keep cleaning equipment handy For example, glass and toilet cleaners in the bathroom. If you're already in there, it makes it that much easier.

Get a Dustbuster Quick tidy-ups make the house look so much better, and your carpets and floors will last longer.

 CALL IN THE PROFESSIONALS. The bad news is that some jobs should be done once a year to keep things safe and up to scratch. The good news is that you don't have to do them. Call in professionals to wash windows, clean flyscreens, shampoo carpets, have upholstered furniture and curtains cleaned, clear out gutters (or better still, have those wire strainers installed), clean paths and remove moss.

Burglar-proof your home

An astonishing number of burglaries occur because people simply forget to lock doors and windows. There are several things you should do to protect your home from a crook who's looking for an easy mark:

Lock all doors and windows Make it a habit to check that doors and windows are locked last thing at night and before you leave the house in the morning. Install deadlocks on doors and windows.

Jam sliding doors Place a length of dowelling or a broom handle in the track of a sliding door so it can't be slid open, even if the lock is jemmied open.

Secure doors near glass If there's a pane of glass next to or in your front door, consider getting a lock that can only be opened from the inside with a key (and don't leave the key dangling there).

Plant prickly shrubs under your windows to create a physical barrier

Install movement detector lights outside You should especially do this in backyards and down side paths.

Put security bars on vulnerable side windows

Join or start a neighbourhood watch group According to police statistics, vigilant neighbours remain the greatest deterrent to crime.

If you're going away, don't shut all the curtains Instead, arrange a house-sitter or ask a neighbour to come in and out regularly, turning lights off and on and opening and shutting curtains. Or buy timer lights and put them in different rooms so they can be seen both from the street and the backyard. Do not leave a message on your answering machine that indicates you're away. Make sure that any ladders or outdoor furniture that could be used to gain access to your home are locked away. Leave the radio on.

Invest in an electronic home security system Look for one that is simple to use, kid-friendly, offers a decent warranty period and has, ideally, a 24-hour call-out repair service.

 KEEP THINGS OUT OF SIGHT. Don't put expensive sound equipment, or other valuable items like computers, near windows where they can easily be seen.

Prevent accidents

Advice to children crossing the street: damn the lights. Watch the cars. The lights ain't never killed nobody.

MOMS MABLEY, ACTIVIST AND WRITER

You're four times more likely to be injured in an accident at home than in work- and car-related accidents combined. Here's how to reduce your risk:

Avoid falls Secure carpet edges and put non-slip mats under rugs. Run electrical and telephone cords along walls. Pick up clutter – toys are the worst offenders for tripping people up. Wipe up anything you've spilled on the floor straightaway. Put rubber mats in showers and baths, and install hand grips. Make sure all staircases have secure handrails. Put nightlights near bedrooms and bathrooms, and check all staircases and walkways are well lit.

Reduce the risk of poisoning Lock all medicines in a secure box where children can't reach them. Store household cleaners in a lockable cupboard. Never leave small children unattended in a garage, bathroom or kitchen. Never store poisonous substances, e.g. methylated spirits, in recycled food or drink containers.

Install smoke detectors – at least one on each floor Change the batteries twice a year. Make sure everyone in the household understands what to do in a fire. Organise a fire drill and get everyone to join in. Keep at least two fire extinguishers – one in the kitchen, and one at the other end of the house. Check them regularly and replace them when they expire.

Make sure you have electrical circuit breakers They are mandatory in all new homes. If you live in an older style house or flat, ask an electrician to install them – they help prevent death or injury from electrocution by instantly shutting off the power if any plugged-in appliance overheats or comes in contact with water.

Buy safety goggles They are vital for avoiding eye injury in many everyday tasks, e.g. lawn mowing.

 GET A STRONG, LIGHTWEIGHT LADDER. Keep it in a convenient spot to reduce the chances of someone clambering up on a chair or other unsuitable surface because they're in a hurry.

Cleaning your house while your kids are still growing is like shovelling the path before it stops snowing.

PHYLLIS DILLER, COMEDIENNE AND ACTRESS

Child-proof your house

I love children, and nearly always have some small friend with me – a godchild, a neighbour – as well as my sons and all their friends. Even if your children have left home and you only have other people's children occasionally visit your home, it's wise to recognise and correct safety risks, so that you can maintain your sanity when they come to visit. The following safety precautions are essential:

Cover exposed power points with plastic safety shields Tie electrical cords together and tape them down along skirting boards to prevent tripping.

Keep curtain and blind cords out of children's reach

Secure cabinet doors Put a childproof latch or lock on cabinet doors that contain household cleaners or other toxic substances, e.g. under-sink cupboards in the kitchen and bathroom and medicine chests. Lock glass-fronted display cabinets and put the key out of reach, rather than leave it in the door.

Keep plastic bags out of children's reach Put them somewhere like the top shelf of a linen press or kitchen cupboard.

Keep any decks or balconies off limits This is important as tiny bodies can easily slip through railings.

Lock any upstairs windows or screens

Block staircases and driveways Put a safety gate or other sturdy blockade at the top and bottom of staircases, and across driveways or paths that lead to the street.

Secure top-heavy furniture You can do this by plugging items (such as bookcases) to the wall with inexpensive safety angle-arms, available at any hardware store.

 REMOVE ORNAMENTAL DISHES containing nuts, small sweets, buttons, toys or ornaments that may be choking hazards This is also wise if you have pets, especially dogs.

Choose hardy house plants

Perennials are the ones that grow like weeds, biennials are the ones that die this year instead of next, and hardy annuals are the ones that never come up at all.

KATHARINE WHITEHORN, COMEDIENNE

Placing a few plants around can cheer up any room immediately, but if you always seem to kill them, perhaps you're choosing the wrong ones. Here are a few suggestions for plants that actually like to be ignored:

Aloe (*Aloe barbadensis*) Nicknamed 'the medicine plant' because of its traditional use for soothing skin problems, especially healing burns, this graceful succulent looks good in a kitchen. Being a member of the cactus family, aloe is about as low maintenance as they come, but it does need reasonable light.

Cast iron plant (*Aspidistra elatior*) This plant's name should give hope to even the brownest of thumbs. Hugely popular in Victorian parlours, it has long, dark-green, spear-shaped leaves. With light and fertiliser it will grow quite big, and works well as a display on a stand.

Chinese evergreen (*Aglaonema* 'Silver Queen') An appealing plant with pretty, silvery, pointed leaves, it prefers filtered light and hates draughts, so it's excellent for perking up dim corners.

Ficus (*Ficus benjamina*) Also known as the weeping fig, this graceful plant needs reasonable light, moderate water and regular fertilising – wedge one of those fertiliser stakes in the pot's soil to help you remember.

Snake plant (*Sanseviera trifasciata*) This virtually indestructible plant got its name thanks to its long, sharp, upward-stretching leaves. Like its cactus cousins, it does best when kept fairly dry and it needs plenty of light.

 GRAB SOME GREEN. Practitioners of feng shui (an Eastern discipline that purportedly helps you finetune your environment for comfort and success) believe plants increase vitality, which is the first step towards achieving happiness.

Bathroom storage solutions

Old medicines, half-used jars of face cream, bandages, cotton wool, sunscreen, plastic bath toys: they're all there, lurking in the bathroom cabinet. The bathroom should be a place where you can refresh and restore yourself, so get rid of anything that doesn't support this objective. Here's how:

Create extra space Utilise walls to hang extra shelves, or buy wicker or mesh stackable baskets or trays for towels, toilet paper and toiletries. Under-sink wheeled trolleys, pegs and hooks are options for even the smallest bathroom.

Install enough towel rails for everyone's towel A heated towel rail is a yummy luxury on a winter morning. It also helps towels dry quicker and reduces damp, musty smells.

Toss out expired medicines Store all drugs and medical supplies in a lockable first aid box.

Discard old toiletries and fragrances This is especially important if they're over a year old. Unopened fragrant products, such as aftershave and cologne, should last about two years, but if they've been opened or exposed to light, the formula oxidises and breaks down. The shelf life of moisturisers, suntan lotion, toothpaste and shampoo is usually between two and three years, but this also decreases once opened. Cosmetics with less water in them (lipstick) will last longer than those with more (body lotions). Items mixed with saliva, such as mouthwashes or eye cosmetics, will go off quickest of all. Signs of decay include rancid odour, oil separation, flaking and discolouration.

Group similar items For example, put hair preparations together and bath items together. Take into account what order you use the different items in, and how often. For instance, if you only style your hair every two or three days, store gels and sprays behind the more frequently-used items, such as toothbrush and toothpaste.

MONITOR ITEMS FOR YOUR SHOPPING LIST. Get into the habit of noticing how much of something is left – especially frequently-used items such as toilet paper, toothpaste, soap, shampoo or tissues – and put it on the shopping list before you run out.

Have a first aid kit handy

Either buy a first aid kit from the chemist, or assemble your own. If you have small children, you must store it well out of their reach. Check your kit every few months and replace any missing or expired items. Here's a selection of what you need:

first aid manual

fever and/or pain relievers e.g. aspirin, paracetamol

antibiotic cream for cuts and scrapes

disinfectant liquid for cleaning wounds

decongestants and cough syrup and/or lozenges

indigestion tablets

adhesive bandages in several sizes and shapes

tweezers

thermometer

cotton balls, sterile gauze pads and rolls of gauze for wrapping wounds

scissors

elastic bandage

safety pins and a length of calico or cotton for making slings

saline eye drops and an eye bath

a medicine measuring glass or dropper

an icepack for sprains and bruises – keep it in the freezer

 GET TWO FIRST AID KITS. Every home should have one kit in the house and one in the car.

Get a grip on the garage

You mightn't have a garage, but chances are you have a shed, cellar or storage room that you try not to think about. The problem with this sort of area is that it's a place to keep the car, a rainy day play area for kids, as well as being a storage area for all sorts of things that don't or won't go in the house. So, the first question is: what is this area's main purpose? This will help you decide what needs to be thrown out or kept elsewhere, and how the things that remain should be arranged. Here's how:

Toss as much as possible Take everything out, tackling the area wall by wall, section by section. If that old golf buggy has a broken handle, ask yourself if you're ever going to fix it – if not, put it aside for the tip. Group things that are staying with other like objects.

Clean up as you go Sweep the floor and wipe down shelves and sills. In a garage, hose the floor and let it dry before you put things back.

Create storage Shelves or adjustable racking can hold boxes, paints and bottles. Pre-holed particle board with hooks is great for hanging tools. Use ceiling racks or a net for large, infrequently used items such as fishing rods and camping equipment.

Get the right tools Throw out anything that's broken, rusty or loose. Most hardware stores sell ready-made toolboxes, some already stocked with basic tools. The minimum it should contain is fuse wire, a hacksaw, a hammer, nails (a few different sizes), a paint scraper, paintbrushes, pliers, a retractable steel tape measure (at least 3 metres long), screwdrivers (various sizes, including a Phillips one), screws, an adjustable spanner, a Stanley knife and string. Also handy are picture hangers, a glue gun, superglue, a putty knife and hole-filling compound, thumbtacks, duct and masking tape and electrical tape.

Get the right gardening equipment Here is a basic check list: edge-trimmer and lawnmower (unless you have a regular garden service); secateurs and shears; bamboo leaf rake; gardening gloves; rubber boots or gardening clogs; fork and spade; trowel – you may want a narrow one for weeding and a broader one for digging out flowers and seedlings. And, it goes without saying, a light straw hat.

 MAINTAIN TOOLS PROPERLY. They're expensive and will last a lot longer with commonsense care. Wipe down tools after use, as even a light film of moisture will cause them to rust. Your hardware store can give you the name of someone who will sharpen lawnmower blades, saws and secateurs.

Freud is all nonsense. The secret of neurosis is to be found in the family battle of wills to see who can refuse the longest to wipe down the bathroom sink. The bathroom sink is the great symbol of the bloodiness of family life.

NORA EPHRON, AUTHOR

Make your kitchen work harder

Your kitchen probably has a number of flaws, but there's a lot you can do to make it more efficient. Here's how:

De-clutter cupboards Throw away broken or chipped crockery and recycle what you no longer like or use; check use-by dates and discard and replace outdated food.

Store like with like For example, put all the glasses or canned goods together. Or, store items together that aren't alike but which are used together, such as everything you use when you barbecue.

Consider frequency of use Match things you use most often (such as salt and pepper, sugar, tea and coffee) with prime storage areas – those spaces that are the most visible and where it's easiest to store or retrieve something.

Keep benchtops clear Avoid arrangements of decorative canisters or baskets, unless they're earning their keep filled with frequently-used items.

Use a ceiling frame They are great for large items such as woks and saucepans. However, if they're not used regularly, they will gather dust.

Utilise wall space Mount electrical appliances, such as microwave ovens, on brackets.

Install baskets, divider racks or turntables If you put them in awkward corners you can avoid losing items at the back of a deep cupboard or shelving. If you have under-bench space, use baskets or plastic boxes to store cake tins.

Keep waste bins behind cupboard doors It's depressing to see overflowing rubbish.

Set up a compost bin This allows you to recycle your food wastes.

Stop smells Store citrus fruits, onions and potatoes in wire or plastic racks to ensure air flow.

Store small items Use flat, low-edged baskets or trays to store small items such as spices.

 LABEL JARS THAT LOOK THE SAME. An easy way to distinguish self-raising flour, plain flour and cornflour is to snip the label off the packet, including the use-by date, and put it into the jar.

Kids' mess

Children. You can't live with them – and you can't live with them.

ROBIN WILLIAMS, COMEDIAN

There are two schools of thought when it comes to kids' rooms: shut the door and never go in, or teach them to keep their rooms organised, fun and bright. Yes, it seems easier to do it yourself, but it's far better to help them gain the competence you hope they'll have when they leave home.

Have a polished floor, if possible It can be easily mopped. Add colourful, washable rugs. To prevent the rugs from slipping, use non-slip matting squares.

Save paintwork Run string lines along the walls so drawings can be pegged up, thus saving wear and tear on paintwork by avoiding the use of Blu Tack or nails.

Set up areas for specific activities Preschoolers need a small table and chair where they can sit to paint, draw or model. Teenagers need a desk with good lighting.

Install adequate shelving Store (while displaying) books, rock collections, Playstation equipment, groups of dolls and bears.

Create storage Have a rubbish basket. Stackable plastic tool or tackle boxes are perfect for organising lots of little things. Make sure containers have clasps that small fingers can negotiate. Buy a multi-purpose bed. Options include: a bed with storage drawers; one that has space for shallow storage bins on wheels; an elevated bed that creates room underneath for a desk or storage; or a trundle bed – one that has another bed underneath that can be pulled out for a friend to sleep over.

Label shelves, drawers and cupboards Use words or, with littlies, pictures.

Come down to their level Little kids have a genuine excuse for not hanging things up – lower rods and hooks to a height that allows them to be reached. As they grow, raise the rods and hooks. Hanging shoe bags on the inside of a wardrobe door keeps them at eye level.

 CULL POSSESSIONS REGULARLY. Once children are over seven or eight, discuss this process with them so they learn to make decisions about what they will need or won't use again. Fix broken toys or throw them away – a broken toy can be dangerous. Give outgrown clothes to friends, family or charity.

Find your keys

My grandfather once told me that there are two kinds of people: those that do the work and those that take the credit. He told me to try to be in the first group; there is much less competition

INDIRA GANDHI, PRIME MINISTER OF INDIA

Eliminate the absolutely unnecessary and exasperating time-wasting experience of searching for your keys. Mount a screw-in hook (or hooks, if everyone else in the family has problems with keys too) in a spot you can't avoid when you are coming into or going out of the house with your keys in your hand. For most people, that's the front hall, but it might be the side door that leads to the kitchen, or just inside the laundry. If your hook is going to withstand daily assaults, it's got to be pretty solid. Most gift and craft shops carry attractive wooden plaques with hooks for hanging keys. You're bound to find a style you like. Consciously develop the habit of using the hook and it will eventually become second nature.

GET AT LEAST ONE EXTRA SET OF KEYS CUT and keep them somewhere safe. You only need lock yourself out of your home or car once to realise what a costly and time-consuming process hiring a locksmith is!

Is your fridge a health hazard?

When it comes to health, I recommend frequent doses of that rare commodity – common sense.

DR VINCENT ASKEY, PAST PRESIDENT, AMERICAN MEDICAL ASSOCIATION

Badly stored food can harbour a formidable range of disease-causing bugs. Stay safe and keep your fridge well-stocked, clean and pleasant to use with these tips:

Invest in a good quality frost-free fridge You won't have to defrost it.

Put a small bowl of vanilla essence on the back shelf This gives it a nice smell.

Don't jam food in Allow airflow between items. You should be able to see what's at the back. If you can't, it's time for a clean out.

Wrap meat, chicken and fish in plastic wrap Then place on a plate to prevent them dripping on other foods.

Keep fruit and vegetables in the crisper drawers Wipe the drawers out regularly.

Store strong-smelling salamis and cheese in airtight containers This way their smell won't taint other food.

Label the container Write the name of the dish and the date prepared on the container before freezing meals you've prepared in advance.

Don't thaw food on a bench or sink, or under hot water Thaw or marinate meat in the bottom of the fridge or, if you need it quickly, in the microwave.

Clean up spills quickly Otherwise, the stickiness seems to spread to everything else in the fridge. You should especially do this if fruit juice lands on the fridge seal as this makes it prone to splitting.

Close the fridge door after use Even just briefly opening it will cause the fridge temperature regulator to readjust as cold air escapes quickly, the re-cooling wastes electricity and costs you money. Encourage everyone to close the door – especially teenage boys who are the worst offenders!

 DISCARD LEFTOVERS AFTER TWO DAYS. Moulds and bacteria develop rapidly. Don't rely on the 'sniff test' – while it's a good measure of edibility, it doesn't ensure safety. When in doubt, throw it out.

Stock up

To ensure things in your kitchen run smoothly, make sure you have the basic tools, equipment and ingredients:

Knives The bare minimum is one small paring knife, one all-purpose knife, and one serrated knife for slicing bread.

Cooking equipment You should have a vegetable peeler, cutting boards, saucepans, at least two frypans, a heavy lidded casserole for making soup, toaster, grater, colander, mixing bowls, baking pan, can opener, salt and pepper grinders, measuring cups, measuring spoons, utensils (such as wooden spoons, soup ladle, tongs, spatula, potato masher, mallet, egg slice, mesh strainer and whisk), oven thermometer, kettle, plastic containers, tea towels, sponges and pot-holders. Also nice to have are a coffee grinder and maker, large salad bowls, salad spinner, hand-held electric mixer, sharpening steel and vegetable steamer.

In the pantry You will always be able to make a quick and easy meal if you have the right ingredients on hand. A basic shopping list should include olive oil, vegetable oil, vinegar, mustard, garlic, soy sauce, tea and coffee, dried herbs (oregano, basil, thyme, rosemary are the most versatile), salt and pepper, canned beans, pasta (at least one long and one short variety), nuts (pecans, pine nuts and peanuts), couscous, rice, bottled pasta sauce, canned or bottled essentials (such as olives, tomatoes, raisins, marinated artichoke hearts, mushrooms, tuna, salmon and corn), stock (cubes or packet base), onions and potatoes.

Fridge basics Your fridge should contain eggs, butter or margarine, plain yoghurt, Parmesan cheese and carrots. Always keep spare bread and rolls, sausages, frozen vegetables and chicken breasts in the freezer.

 BUY THE BEST KNIVES YOU CAN AFFORD. Cheaper ones are often a false economy as they dull easily and aren't always sturdy enough to last the distance.

Take an inventory

Housekeeping ain't no joke.

LOUISA MAY ALCOTT, AUTHOR

Agreed, making an inventory is not the most relaxing task. However, once it's done, you only have to update it now and then. And, in the hopefully unlikely event of burglary or property damage, at least you'll be able to put your hands on all the right documentation to support your insurance claim. Here's how to get started:

Make a list Take a clipboard and pen and go from room to room, noting furniture along with all other contents, e.g. paintings, curtains, rugs, ornaments, toys, electrical equipment and tools. Where possible, especially with whitegoods, note the brand, model and serial numbers.

Take photos It's a good idea to use a video camera to document each room or area – as you slowly pan around the room, talk about particular items, and open cupboards and drawers to show what's in them. Or photograph everything as you go around with the list.

Include everyday items An inventory should cover everything in your home, from the most to the least expensive – the cat litter tray, sewing machine, frying pan and iron are just as important as your pearls and good leather handbags. Make sure you take in the garage, cellar, attic and garden areas. Include items such as outdoor furniture, lawnmower and car-related supplies.

Have valuables appraised Take special items to a jeweller to be professionally valued. Enlist the services of a qualified valuer to provide an appraisal on stamp or coin collections, silverware, antiques, rugs or pieces of art. Photograph them and attach the picture to the relevant certificates.

Keep it safe When you've finished (phew!), make copies. Keep one with all relevant receipts, appraisals and photos at an independent location. It's also wise to leave at least one other copy with a close friend or relative.

 UPDATE YOUR INVENTORY. Each time you purchase something new for your home, get into the habit of adding it to the list, along with the receipt and details.

Planning essentials
The household useful box

Every home should have one – a container, box or dish, which contains all those bits
and pieces that people are always wasting time looking for. 'Mum, have you seen the
sticky tape?' 'Dear, are there any batteries?' Go through it regularly and toss out the
take away menus and collectables from chip packets that also seem to end up there.
My 'useful box' is on top of the fridge, and it contains:

stamps

candles plus appropriate holders, in case of a power blackout

batteries including several sizes for torches, Gameboys, clocks and so on

a torch that works

rubber bands

emergency tool kit including a tiny screwdriver for fixing hinges on arms of
glasses, and fuse wire

twist-ties for plastic bags

extension cord

band aids

matches

pens

pencils, rubber and sharpener

electrical double adapter

spare light globes

string

The kids' useful box

Chez Allardice has tackled some amazingly involved school projects: making a scale model of a goldmine; making an agricultural irrigation system and making a model of the human urinary system (no I am not making this up). I found out about each one at dinnertime the night before it was due. My hard-won, through-gritted-teeth-solution is to have a second useful box, exclusively for kids' school projects. It should be large, have a lid (so you don't have to look at the junk inside) and be kept out of sight so it can't be ransacked by kids for ordinary play, leaving you to make a wild-eyed dash to a hideously expensive 24-hour supermarket. You need:

tissues (snow, surf, dresses, child's tears)

felt scraps (grass, mountains, paddocks)

styrofoam balls (just dandy for planets)

cottonwool and/or cottonwool balls (clouds, and anything to do with Christmas)

ice-cream sticks (mine shafts, buildings, oars, bridges, fences)

cotton reels (turrets, wheels, drums)

empty matchboxes (drawers, steps, beds, wardrobes, trucks)

old used-up biros (boat masts, pylons, spears)

cellophane (red for fire or volcano lava, clear for all sorts of other things)

foil (lakes, machinery, money)

egg cartons

shoe boxes, plus extra shoebox lids (as bases)

old containers (ice-cream or margarine are versatile)

old costume jewellery (brilliant when I had to make Davy Jones' locker for an 'under the sea' project)

odds and sods for creating realistic-looking machinery (old watch or clock workings are useful) and there are always uses for feathers, rocks and pebbles, pipe cleaners, straws, old screw-top bottle caps and balloons

stuff to keep it all together so it survives the trip on the way to school – fuse wire, Blu Tack, superglue, spray adhesive, sticky tape, duct or masking tape

I think that people are just about as happy as they make up their minds to be.

ABRAHAM LINCOLN

Feed the spirit

Be present in the moment

Don't get so busy with the physical running of a home and children that you miss the glory of rearing a family, just as the grandeur of the trees is lost when raking leaves.

MARCELENE COX

When you are truly focussed, you find more satisfaction in everyday life. Being truly focussed means that you direct all your energy into whatever you're doing. Even if you're sitting on a park bench, you still try to accord importance to those minutes of relaxation, soaking up your surroundings with all your senses. Such moments are an antidote for the rest of your hectic life, but learning to do it isn't easy. You need to become more flexible and take each step more deliberately. You need to stay open to unexpected changes in the day's emotional weather and respond accordingly, so you fully inhabit your life from one moment to the next. You need to make your peace with slow-moving or unplanned events: a dirty kitchen floor, unexpected interruptions, a delay or strike. Here's how:

Make two small changes every day Take a different street, try a new cafe, change your toothpaste, smile at someone you don't know. There's a lot of landscape to explore off the beaten path.

Take a TV-fast A recent poll showed that, in the average household, the TV is on for a minimum of 50 hours a week. Much of that time is spent watching whatever's on rather than a specific, interesting program. If you're a habitual TV watcher, and want to discover simple pleasures as a way to relax, try fasting from TV. Time will simply open up.

Realise not everything needs to be done today Prioritise what feels right, not just what your to-do list says. If the day's rhythm favours cleaning rather than returning phone calls, that's what should get done. Tasks will still get taken care of, but the doing of them will flow better and you'll feel more peaceful.

 CHOOSE STILLNESS over activity. Choose being over doing. Let go of the impossible and embrace what is right there in front of you, right this minute.

Pamper yourself

There must be quite a few things in life that a hot bath won't cure, but I don't know many of them.

SYLVIA PLATH, AUTHOR AND POET

Pick your favourite treatments, or – better yet – try them all:

Take an Epsom salts bath It's an inexpensive way to make your skin feel much smoother. Add 2 cups of salts and 4–6 drops of essential oil: lavender has a calming effect, lemon will awaken your senses.

Scrub up Mix together 1 cup oatmeal, 2 teaspoons each of honey, olive oil and powdered milk, $1/2$ cup water, and 3 tablespoons of Epsom salts. Apply to damp skin (avoiding eye area, and working very gently round sensitive areas like nipples) and then rinse. Finish with a thick body lotion.

Steam your face Boil 4 cups of water, pour it into a heat-resistant bowl, and add 3–5 drops of a calming essential oil, such as rose or ylang ylang. Cover your head with a towel and let the steam envelop your face for 10 minutes.

Get glowing A self-tanner is a smart way to get a healthy glow without too much sun.

Add colour to how you look and feel Try a new hair colour, a tinted moisturiser, and some lip and cheek colour.

Beat bad hair After shampooing, rinse with a 50:50 mixture of warm water and apple cider vinegar. It reduces frizz and also removes dirt, mineral deposits and soapy residue.

 ADD CUCUMBER SLICES to your water jug. This spa trick makes those eight glasses of water a day even more palatable and beneficial, as studies have found that cucumber's fresh scent and taste reduce anxiety.

Ditch emotional baggage

*If you can't get rid of the skeletons in your closet,
at least teach them to dance.*

GEORGE BERNARD SHAW

Just as too much alcohol, nicotine, or rich or processed foods make our bodies sluggish, our mind gets clogged up over the years with limiting, stressful, and often unjustified beliefs. This is known as emotional baggage. Here are some steps to take towards dumping yours:

Acknowledge emotional black spots There are certain feelings we always push to the back of our minds – especially fear, whether it's of change or of heights. If fear is stopping you doing things you'd like to do, acknowledging that it's there is the first step. However painful your feelings, it's better to get them out in the open. Only then can you work out ways of overcoming the fear, perhaps with the help of a therapist.

Break the pattern If something feels comfortable, it's natural to do it over and over again, but sometimes the reason it feels pleasant is because it's familiar, not because it's right or best for you. Think about why you've made certain choices and whether they were good ones. Career and relationship mistakes are almost always made when you choose the sort of option you think you ought to, rather than the one you want to.

Give yourself a break You can't make everyone in your life happy all the time. And it's OK to make mistakes now and then.

 LIKE YOURSELF. Don't try to be perfect. Learning to accept yourself as you are sets you free. It also lets others be themselves in your presence and that makes you good company.

Tune into nature

I go to nature to be soothed and healed,
and to have my senses put in order.

JOHN BURROUGHS, WRITER

Spending even just a few minutes outdoors each day can have a profound effect on both your psyche and your health. Nature provides many things we need, such as fresh air and sunshine, but there's also an energy in living things that feeds our spirit; we realise that we're just one of many species, and that we're connected to other forms of life. Try the following ideas:

Ask yourself, 'Can I do this outside?' Doing paperwork and reading in the garden or on a sunny terrace can be extremely productive, especially if you're trying to stimulate creativity.

Be adventurous Don't worry about the weather. Wear rain gear or warm clothes. All weather can be enjoyable.

Utilise plants and windows They are vital for city dwellers and people who can't get outside easily. Just looking at a tree outside your window for a few moments can make you feel better.

Use full-spectrum light bulbs They mimic sunlight and you can buy them in most health food and home improvement stores.

Appreciate details Next time you're relaxing in a grassy area, lie on your stomach or side and examine the blades of grass, noting their colour and texture. Take a tour of your backyard or nearest park and notice the various types of trees. Do you know what kind each one is? If not, bring a guide to trees with you next time.

✳ NOTICE NATURE. For many people, nature is an abiding source of inspiration.

Unravel with 'the new yoga'

My problem is I internalise everything. I don't relax when I'm stressed; I grow a tumour instead.

WOODY ALLEN

Once considered an activity for seniors or back-to-earth types, knitting has become the latest way to relax. Finding comfort in stressful times, creating handmade treasures to pass on to loved ones: these are the threads that weave together knitting's past, present and future. Knitting's calming effects come from the repetitive rhythms of needles, yarn and hands, a combination that induces the classic 'relaxation response', marked by lowered heart rate and blood pressure. In fact, any kind of repetitive activity, whether it's reciting a rosary or power walking, can induce this meditative state in the brain. Unlike ordinary rest, meditation increases both mental alertness and relaxation.

You don't have to learn fancy techniques or invest in expensive equipment to get started. Here's how you can get into the stitch of things:

Visit your local craft or wool shop, or stitchery Employees are usually terrific sewers or knitters and can guide you about what you need, especially if you're a beginner.

Start with the basics Anyone who knows how to knit can teach you the basic plain-and-purl rhythm or simple embroidery stitches. Start on something easy – a knitted scarf, for instance, or a cross-stitch sampler.

Join a group Most craft or wool shops offer beginners' classes or can point you in the direction of a local group. Perhaps most importantly, such groups bring together women of all backgrounds, providing the kind of support they don't always get in their daily lives.

TAKE UP A HOBBY. Do something for the sheer pleasure of it – whether it's knitting, collecting rocks or birdwatching. Hobbies help instill self-confidence and often connect you with others who share your interests. And being engaged in numerous pursuits will help shield you from depression.

Add meaning to your life

Our complex lives don't just stress us out, they distract us from what's really important. While you might have experienced an increase in material affluence, there could also be a gnawing sense that such gains won't satisfy the deeper parts of your being. Here's how to enhance your spiritual life:

Connect with your heritage Whether your background is Christian, Buddhist or Muslim, building bridges to your past culture can bring depth and meaning to your life. It might, for instance, result in an interest in Celtic mythology, or perhaps improvising children's prayers that blend both formal and personal beliefs. Understanding your heritage shows that you are part of something much larger – a spiritual world.

Stretch your body, focus your mind Yoga gives a wonderful feeling of groundedness and connection: in the practice of yoga, the intention, classically, is to unite the individual soul with the universal soul. There is a sense of maintaining complete wellbeing, beyond the physical aspects of just trying to look good. Yoga takes you to a state of deep quiet, focussing your awareness and concentration.

Find a community You don't necessarily have to turn to organised religion: spiritual seekers can sign up for silent retreats, or for classes in meditation, qigong, rebirthing, life after death, astrology, tarot, Sufi dancing, chanting, sacred drumming, shamanism – all have their adherents. People's images of God vary enormously – the 'right' one is the one that is personal, intimate and authentic for you.

Do good deeds For many, finding spiritual satisfaction may boil down to plain, old-fashioned helping others – volunteering at a soup kitchen, tutoring a teenager, reading to patients in a hospice – so that life is not all about me, me, me.

 CULTIVATE KINDNESS wherever you can. Tell the checkout operator in the supermarket that you appreciate the way your groceries are packed so that the tomatoes aren't squashed. Call or visit a housebound friend. Bake a cake for the kids next door. Giving raises your self-worth and connects you to others.

Pets keep you positive

One of the hardest things about working in the health care industry, as I do, is putting up with the steady stream of bad news pumped out by researchers. Popcorn is bad for you (coconut oil). Biscuits are bad for you (trans fatty acids). Your beef's got antibiotics in it, not to mention how they farm chickens these days. And I won't even start on water.

This is why it is such a joy to find things we like that are actually good for us. Take chocolate, for instance. Recently scientists have shown that it raises your 'good' cholesterol. Even taking risks – just the opposite of what a sensible person thinks he or she ought to do – has been shown to help stabilise a stress-filled life. However, nothing compares with the research into the effects of owning pets. For a pittance in food I can lower my blood pressure, improve my mood, and up my chances of surviving a heart attack.

It shouldn't surprise me, I guess. I may have forgotten the names and faces of people I went to school with but I will never forget Thaddeus, my mother's enormous grey Persian cat, standing up and putting her paws on Mum's chin then gently head-butting her when she came back to the house after Dad's funeral. Or Sandy, our other family cat, who used to hide behind the fence, ambush the labrador next door, and hold on majestically for an invigorating, ears-flat-back ride as the dog tore back and forth trying to dislodge its passenger. Or Orange the goldfish, Cherish the canary, Lucky the mouse (so named because one of the cats spat him out), Bambi, Bo Bo, Pyewacket, Boadicea the Warrior Queen, Amonetta, Yum Yum, Petal, Barnstaple, Sabine, Maxima, Tom and Ian – the last three of whom are circling my ankles as I write, waiting for me to walk to the kitchen so that for the thousandth time they can come up and declare with every passionate rub and purr, 'God, it's about time. We're so glad you're home'.

 THEY'RE WORTH IT. Our animal friends keep primed the open-hearted side of all of us. Regrettably, they don't live forever, and I have buried many beloved pets after illness or accident. But ask any pet owner and they'll tell you the heartache is worth it. Besides, I now know that in exchange for every flea bath I've given, every cage I've cleaned and every meal I've dished up, I've added hours to my life.

Those whose work and pleasure are found in the same place are fortune's favourite children.

WINSTON CHURCHILL

Out of the mouths of babes

I know it's a hopeless cliché, but as a mum I find I learn a lot of very important things from my kids. How to be curious and interested in everyday things, for instance. ('What's this, Mummy?' 'Moss, darling.' 'It's like a fairy pillow, Mum.') Or how to make really good hide-outs. Or how to throw a serious tantrum. Or (here comes another cliché) how to have the right attitude when faced with adversity.

This was brought home to me most succinctly by Randall when he was about five. A sturdy, rosy-faced little boy with a serious blue gaze and few words, Randall had always seemed to have a deceptively simplistic view of the world. If he'd had a good day at kindergarten and liked what I was making for dinner, you could ask him how he was and he'd say, 'Great'. (Well, honesty demands that I tell you that he actually said 'Gate'. He wasn't too good on Rs.) Anyway, if things weren't going quite the way he wanted them to, and you asked the same question, he'd answer with a frown of concentration, a patient sigh, and 'Not gate yet'.

When you think about the frantic way we try to live these days – never seeming to have enough time for what we think we really want, watching the clock, worrying that our jobs are taking over our lives or that we're becoming slaves to our possessions – I still think Randall's answer is quite refreshing, really.

LEARN FROM CHILDREN'S WISDOM. No matter how rough or crazy the road seems at the moment, we can all be reasonably sure that we're on the way to 'gate', even if we're not there yet.

On balance

A sense of balance is an important tool to have in your back pocket. I have found myself thinking lately of the many ways in which our minds and lives teeter on the edges of ideas, habits, values – how every day and every decision is a balancing act.

We balance our time between work and family – between the need to excel and the need to relax. We balance our meals and our diets and move the meat to the side to make room for more vegetables and fruit and pasta. We balance our chequebooks. (Well, we try to.) We balance our attitudes between being satisfied with what we've done and wanting to do better. We try to be tolerant of differences and open to new ideas while holding on to what we value. We maintain a respect for history and memories of Grandma's wisdom while we discover new ways of doing things, of working towards greater efficiencies, and of coping with the technology that is all-pervasive in our lives. We weigh up lessons we've learned in the past against the promises that lie ahead. We value accuracy and truth and facts, while we continue to look for beauty, grace and symmetry.

Obligations, deadlines and stress stretch along the corridors of our lives like tightropes. But it's so important to counterbalance all this calculated balancing we do – to consciously aim for a sense of equilibrium, to relax, to celebrate, to spend time with our families and friends, to eat splendid meals and to indulge.

REMEMBER TO RELAX. As you balance things in your life, don't forget to enjoy yourself. This is why I wish you warmth, health and happiness – and a little joyful excess – to balance the equation.

A positive perspective

A while back, my cousin Elizabeth fell off the roof and broke her arm. Then she got fired. But she didn't get depressed. 'When bad things happen', she says, 'I think about them – then I figure out what I'm going to do next.' I, on the other hand, come from a long line of people with half-empty cups who are always looking on the glum side. I may not be as optimistic as Liz, but I'm working on making small changes to my outlook – not automatically assuming, for example, that if I go away on holiday the house will get robbed. Even if you've been raised to be realistic (read: pessimistic) it is possible to learn to see the bright side:

Focus on your strengths as well as your weaknesses Think about positive emotions and events – such as happiness, joy, fun and hope – and take note of what's bad, dangerous, destructive or wrong about ourselves or others. That's being realistic *and* positive.

Be kind to yourself Treating yourself to rewards – a bunch of flowers, theatre tickets, reading the whole newspaper over a leisurely coffee – is not being indulgent, it's necessary to achieving a sense of control over your life.

Reframing is a basic technique favoured by psychologists The trick is to find something – anything – positive in a dreadful situation. Say you got fired. Well, maybe spending more time with your kids for a little while will be a good thing for you and for them.

Don't ignore warning signals Like a flashing red light on your car's dashboard, your feelings can alert you to the fact that something is amiss. If you're angry, jealous, frustrated or just plain irritable, it's a sign that you need to take a deep breath and find a way to change directions.

 SURROUND YOURSELF WITH POSITIVE PEOPLE. A negative person is one of the biggest time-wasters there is. An optimistic outlook is contagious.

Follow your hunches

Learning to use your intuition – that gut feeling you get when you instinctively know what to do in a certain situation – can help you make better decisions about almost everything in your life. Here are some tips for flexing your intuitive muscle:

Get calm If you can't meditate, at least do some relaxation exercises, take a long walk, work in the garden or just retreat to a private room. Anything that quiets the mind will help.

Get creative Look at a geometrical object or pattern, or listen to music that doesn't have words. These stimuli engage the right 'creative' side of your brain and help quiet the left, 'analytical' side.

Play with your intuition Try to guess what someone will be wearing tomorrow, or which is the quickest line at the bank, or which level of the carpark has the best space for you.

Keep a log of intuitive hunches Record how you got them, where you were and what you were doing so you can better understand the patterns of your type of intuition.

Stay neutral Beware of emotional interference such as wishful thinking, which can sabotage your attempts. Stay as neutral as possible.

Lighten up Too much effort backfires, while laughter and fun help ideas and intuition flow more easily.

 AVOID EXPECTATIONS about your intuition. It will present itself in different ways for different people. Some people 'see' things or 'hear' ideas being spoken to them; others notice different or unusual feelings in their bodies.

Turn obstacles into opportunities

The people I'm furious with are the feminists. They keep getting up on soapboxes and proclaiming that women are brighter than men. It's true, but it should be kept quiet or it ruins the whole racket.

ANITA LOOS, SCREENWRITER

When you face a severe test – such as an illness, a financial upheaval, a relationship breakdown, a defeat, or even a tragedy – it can bring you great peace, because it makes you stop and look deeper within. As daunting as an obstacle may be, it marks a turning point. You are now able to say goodbye to your old life and look for ways to make the new life as positive as possible. Here are some ways to help you find happiness wherever you can:

Nurture your relationship with God or Spirit Prayer and quiet contemplation can give you direction.

Meditate Yoga and tai chi can help you develop mental, spiritual and physical balance so you can cope better with the issues you face, and often retain an underlying sense of rightness. Most people don't realise how much inner strength they have until they consciously develop it.

Rewrite your story No matter how traumatic the event, search for a sense of meaning in your suffering. This may not be immediately obvious, but it could be that the event has made you more compassionate, or that you have discovered the importance of forgiveness, or that you have finally let go of bad things that have happened to you. You are, after all, your own life stories, and how you proceed from now on can allow you to feel joy, energy, and peace in your future.

SEE THE MIRACLE IN EVERY MOMENT. Being grateful for everything life sends your way – not just the good times, but the challenging ones too – allows you to get in touch with your soul, and to appreciate the ecstasy of being alive.

Give something back

Loneliness and the feeling of being unwanted is the most terrible poverty.

MOTHER TERESA OF CALCUTTA

Fitting in volunteer or community service or charity work may seem at odds with the idea of setting aside time for yourself, but everyone wins when you do something worthwhile – compassionate behaviour leads to compassionate attitudes, at work and at home. Be selective, though, and only participate in or contribute to a cause if you believe in its worth and if you are personally enthusiastic.

Don't be swayed by emotion In fact, never give time or money if you're being made to feel pressured, uncomfortable or guilty.

Refuse handouts If you are asked for money by someone knocking at your front door, request literature and assess the cause – and its legitimacy – in your own time.

Steer clear of gifts Avoid fundraising organisations selling sunscreen, chocolates or pens at inflated prices. These items are not usually tax-deductible. Make a donation independently and obtain a receipt.

Ask questions If you select volunteer work or charities whose values reflect and support your own, you will feel better about donating time and money. A childless person may enjoy a deeper sense of satisfaction through sponsoring a World Vision child, for example, while if you and your family are concerned about environmental issues, it may feel more appropriate to give your time on Clean-up Day. Most organisations are only too happy to assist you with any research.

Work to a budget When you put together your financial plan, allocate how much money to donate to charity, then decide who will receive it. Planning ahead will help you achieve your tax and philanthropic goals, as well as help you steer clear of emotive appeals.

 BE CAUTIOUS. Unfortunately there are many dodgy fundraising operations with names deliberately similar to legitimate charities and causes. Get the exact name in writing and make enquiries before committing any funds or precious time.

Planning essentials
The journal

I still have my first diary – a pink zippered folder with a little gold key to lock in all my secrets – complete with texta hearts, exclamation marks and inked-out initials. Reading over my adolescent angst about clothes, teachers and boys causes me to cringe. I'm more proud of the one I kept when the boys were little, about green dinosaur birthday cakes, backyard forts, football, kittens, sleepovers, beach holidays, school projects, and the ultimate compliment of the little bunch of squished flowers, 'You're nice, Mum'. In other diaries I described the rewards and hardships of working three jobs to make ends meet; later still, after years of being alone with two kids, I confided my trepidation at finding a new partner.

A diary is ongoing and forgiving, and it's there for you when things are good, bad or just mooching along. It's the one place you can be quite truthful and where you can grow without being judged. Here's how to get started:

Choose a special book It could be a beautiful journal or, if that's too intimidating, a plain, lined exercise book, or a password-secured document on your computer.

Find somewhere to write that's comfortable It could be your desk, the kitchen table, a favourite chair or your bed at the end of the day.

Set yourself a daily time limit You can take longer, if you like, or less time. But if you haven't written in a diary for a while, you'll need about 15 minutes to really get going. Try to write something every day – the more you do it, the easier it becomes.

Explore your feelings Dig a bit deeper and examine both negative and positive experiences: note how they've made you feel, how they've affected you and what you're going to do about them. And if you're lacking inspiration, finish the sentence, 'I want to. . .' Another trick is to write a pretend letter to someone, and tell them what's on your mind.

Write about your troubles It can keep you healthy, according to a study from the Southern Methodist University in the USA. One group of students wrote about their worries for 20 minutes twice a week, while the others wrote about ordinary events. In the months after, those who wrote about their troubles were half as likely to visit the doctor than the others.

The library

When was the last time you visited your local library? Perhaps you're already aware of what a fantastic resource it is, but if you haven't joined up, there are plenty of reasons why you should. Here are a few:

It's free Whether you want to find out more about possible hobbies and interests for yourself, or you're chasing information for school projects, your library will be able to help. If a particular book or CD isn't to your taste, there are always more available, and you won't have wasted any money.

It's a great place for kids Most libraries are a mine of information on things like finding a maths coach for your child, or sourcing a craft class, holiday-care program, or babysitter. Same goes for older people: they are a terrific resource for all sorts of clubs, special interest groups and newsletters.

It's quiet If there's a library near your work, give yourself a peaceful lunchbreak by going in there to read the daily newspapers or file magazines. The quiet atmosphere is a balm for a too-busy soul.

The services Ask whether your library is linked to other libraries and information resource facilities around the country and overseas. That way, if you're searching for a particular book or magazine, chances are they will be able to initiate a search on your behalf, at no charge or for a minimal cost.

I hate housework. You make the beds, you do the dishes, and six months later you have to start all over again.

JOAN RIVERS, TALK SHOW HOST

Create order

De-junk your life

Clearing away clutter is like putting your house on a diet. These are the best of the many inexpensive time- and space-saving gadgets you can buy:

Tiered shelves These come in different levels and widths so you can see every jar or can without having to rummage – fantastic for the pantry.

A spice rack, shelf or tray I like narrow shelves just to the height and depth of the spice containers, that can be attached inside an eye-level cupboard. Arrange spices alphabetically.

A basket Keep this under the sink for the wet sponge, scrub pad, dishwashing powder or liquid, and brush. Simply getting these items off the counter lifts the look and feel of the whole kitchen.

Drawer dividers In addition to the standard trays for cutlery, there's a wide range of drawer organisers available: use them in a tool drawer to separate screwdrivers, string and tape; in the kids' drawers to keep socks separate; and to make sense of the kitchen drawer that holds the piping bag, cookie cutters, nutcracker, and all those other awkwardly-shaped bits and pieces.

A shower caddy Hang one over the shower head to organise shampoos, conditioners, soaps and razors that otherwise clutter up the floor of the shower or topple over and leak.

Extra shelves Check the cupboards and wardrobes you have now. Often you will find that there is wasted storage space above the existing top shelf. Have an extra one installed for items you rarely use, such as Christmas tree decorations.

Lots of hooks Put them on the inside of the wardrobe doors for a belt you use every day, on the back of the bathroom door for your dressing gown, or on the kids' bedroom walls for raincoats, school bags and sports equipment.

 AVOID CLUTTER. Busy people often drown themselves in clutter. Such chaos can amplify stress, especially if important things keep vanishing. Spend a little time each day getting rid of superfluous stuff. As a rule, if you haven't used it in a year, you don't need it.

Beat hoarder's disorder

There's an abundance of opportunities to acquire things in our lives. Trouble is, it's just not worth it. The price paid is a lifetime of being loaded down by things we wouldn't miss if they were taken away from us, and disused things that ultimately crowd the necessary things we actually use. Here's how to decide what should be tossed out, given away or sold, and what should be kept:

I might need it someday Sure, you might – but what about all the things you've discarded that you've never needed again? Almost everything is replaceable and you could probably get something similar if you really needed it. Ask yourself, 'Do I need this or simply want it?' You should save it when it is the only copy, when replication would be very difficult, when you need to refer to it again and again, or when you are required by law to keep it.

Use it or lose it If you aren't actually using something, why allow it to complicate your home? Give your grown kids' things back to them. The same goes for other people for whom you are storing things.

It's too nice to throw away If it's that nice, give it to someone who will use and appreciate it.

Is it broken? Get rid of anything that's been broken for more than a year – if you haven't fixed it by now, you're not going to.

Skip the sentiment You are not betraying a person if you pass on an object that reminds you of them, or of a special place you've been together. Nor do you have to be ruthlessly unsentimental. Take the middle path. Keep things that give you a sense of genuine joy, not of obligation or guilt.

Take the 30-day test Save the box the stereo, TV, video or Playstation came in for 30 days. If it hasn't broken by then, toss the box. Unless you're planning on moving very soon, never keep the box 'because you'll need it when you move'.

 BEWARE OF GADGETS. Some people just can't resist the latest thingamajig. When thinking about the timesaving properties of a gadget – whether it's an exercise bike or an ice-cream maker – add in the time it takes to earn the money to buy it, to get it out, use it and clean it. Think about where will you store it. Is it worth it?

Sort out the cupboards

You're not alone in dreading this huge job. However, the pay-off – that sense of accomplishment – is hard to beat. Start early in the morning and choose the cupboard, drawer, room or area that's been annoying you the most.

Take five large cardboard boxes or plastic garbage bags Label them: 'Keep', 'Rubbish', 'Belongs Elsewhere', 'Charity' and 'Mend'. Arrange them in a semicircle around the cupboard door.

Empty the cupboard completely That means taking out every single thing, one object at a time. As you remove an item, put it in the appropriate box. For example, the Christmas tree lights that don't work go in 'Rubbish'. Items that are chipped, broken or stained are not what you want in your life. Your son's sleeping bag? It goes in 'Belongs Elsewhere'. It should be put in his room so he won't have to take the house apart like he did before the last school excursion.

Categorise as you go If you are clearing out boxes of household accounts, you will need to sort your 'Keep' file as you go. Make big, simple categories, such as 'Car', 'Children', 'Health', 'Home', 'Insurance', 'Investments' and 'Tax'. If you're clearing out the linen cupboard, the 'Keep' pile should be separate stacks of, say, sheets, towels, tablecloths and beach towels.

Be a benevolent dictator Before you clean out the cupboard, let everyone else know that they're free to come and get any items they want before you start. You'll defeat the entire purpose if you put everything into the 'Belongs Elsewhere' group, because you'll still have the same stuff – just in different parts of the house!

Take each box or bag to where it belongs Do this straightaway. Don't put the 'Charity' one in the garage, because it will stay there. Take it to the local collection centre on the same day, if possible.

Finally, put back what's left in the 'Keep' pile Don't automatically put the contents back in the same way. Group like items together. Try to place things so that you can see everything on the shelf.

 HANDLE THINGS ONCE. Try not to put any item anywhere 'just for now' and keep it in a perpetual holding pattern. As soon as you do, you are setting yourself up to handle it more than once, and at least doubling your workload. What you're really doing is putting off making a decision – and the decision won't be any easier or quicker to make later on.

Prune your collections

It's remarkable the way that inanimate objects reproduce when you're not looking. China animals, paperweights, letter openers, crystal do-dads, little jugs, pots and jars: they are all prime culprits. They all require dusting and cleaning, which is time-consuming. Here are some ideas on how to get your collections under control:

Get rid of all of it If the collection doesn't really mean anything to you, or you don't look at it or work on it anymore, have a garage sale and sell it, or give the entire collection to a charity.

Get rid of some of it Do what gamekeepers call 'culling', where they reduce the size of a herd when there are too many of a species in one area to be supported by the amount of food and water available. In this case, for example, you could reduce the size of your collection by half or two-thirds, and only keep the most beautiful or valuable pieces, which mean the most to you.

Put it behind glass Naturally, if you love your collection, these first two points won't apply to you. But you can still make it much easier to maintain if you invest in a glass display case to stop all the pieces from getting dusty or dirty.

 CREATE ORDER. Without order, spontaneity is actually chaos. When your life is organised, you can shift direction and take advantage of creative opportunities without causing a crisis in another part of your life. Being organised actually means giving yourself more freedom, not less.

Organise important documents

Put all your documents in a place where they are easy for everyone to find without too much sleuthing. Along with the items listed below, these should include vehicle ownership titles and car registration papers; stock certificates; driver's licence; leases; passports; superannuation fund policies; military records; citizenship papers; insurance policies; and education records, for example, diplomas, degrees and academic transcripts. So, which records should you save, and for how long? Here are some tips:

Forever Keep adoption/birth certificates, custody agreements, death certificates, deeds, passports, birth, marriage and divorce papers, wills and health records.

For 6 years Keep bank statements, cheque butts, credit card receipts, tax records and utility bills (if they contribute to tax deductions).

Until you sell the house Keep home improvement records.

4 years past expiry Keep insurance policies and investment records.

3 years after final payment Keep loan or mortgage documents.

For as long as you keep the appliance Keep owner's manuals, warranties and instructions.

KEEP COPIES. Have photocopies made of all important documents, such as marriage and birth certificates and your household inventory. Keep them in a small home safe, or in a safety deposit box at the bank.

Get the laundry under control

Behind every successful woman is a basket of dirty laundry.

SALLY FORTH, CARTOON CHARACTER

Perhaps, like me, you have a malevolent laundry gremlin: how else can you explain the fact the clothes basket is empty at night, and full in the morning? These ideas can help:

Get the biggest and best washing machine and drier you can afford They are quieter, more reliable and more energy-efficient.

Keep cleaning items handy Store bleach, fabric softener, laundry detergent, pegs, stain remover, starch, wool wash and other items on shelves, or buy wicker or mesh storage baskets on wheels so they can be rolled away.

Have two dirty clothes baskets Label one for colours and one for whites. Train household members to dump things in the right basket to save time sorting.

Set load level, fabric cycle and water temperature according to your needs You'll save time as well as money. As a general guide, use hot water for dirty loads; warm water for whites that are not prone to shrinkage; and cold water on permanent press and colours.

Measure detergent Using too much wastes money, plus it leaves a soapy residue that dulls clothes. If your brand doesn't have a scoop, keep a measuring cup nearby.

Toss in a fabric softener sheet when using the drier They're not expensive and they save time by reducing wrinkles and static when laundry has to be folded.

Take care Following care labels keeps clothes looking better for longer. Closing buttons and zippers saves wear and tear by stopping clothes from catching on parts of the machine or each other. Treat stains straightaway. Use a lingerie bag and the gentle cycle for your underwear rather than having to hand wash.

Hang up items that don't require ironing You should do this while they're still slightly damp so they dry wrinkle-free. If you live in a flat or an area prone to wet weather, buy a portable clothes rack that can be wheeled out onto a verandah, or in front of a heater to dry at night.

 CHECK POCKETS! Picking tiny scraps of soggy white tissue off clothes is one of the biggest time-wasters there is.

Label things

There are plenty of things around the home that we neglect to label because we think it's unnecessary – until we try to retrieve them or put them away, that is. Here are some handy tips:

Storage and archive boxes Take your time. Even if you end up with a label that lists *everything* in each box, doing so is still simpler than looking through all of them to find one item.

Food Everything starts to look the same after a week in the freezer. Keep a roll of freezer-safe tape and a marker pen where you keep your freezer wrap. Name the item – for example, 'Drumsticks' or 'Beef Stew' – and add the date it was stored. That way, if you've got more than one of the same item, you'll know which one to use first.

Make it easy for others Consider the teenager putting the peanut butter back on the wrong shelf, or the eight-year-old cramming toys under their bed. Putting labels on the inside of kitchen cupboards will help prevent haphazard storage, especially if you're not the only one unpacking groceries. Tape a list on the inside of the pantry door, paying particular attention to the things the family tends to look for: cereal, sugar, peanut butter, honey, and so on. Of course, the aim of this exercise is not to remind them where things are – they know that already – it's to remind them where to put them back!

Label kids' clothing and underwear This is particularly important if you've got same-sex siblings who are similar sizes. The easiest way is just to write their initials on a collar with a permanent marker. The laundry will be quicker to sort and it means someone other than you could do it!

 BE SPECIFIC. Labelling things, 'Miscellaneous', 'Children's Stuff', '1998' or 'Dad's Papers', will come back to haunt you because you end up going through the entire box in the hope that a particular item might be in it.

*I try to take one day at a time –
but sometimes several days attack
me at once.*

JENNIFER UNLIMITED, COMEDIENNE

Organise the stuff you clean with

Make sure you have all the essential cleaning items at hand to keep things spick-and-span. Here's a basic list to check your supplies against:

broom

buckets

dusters including a chamois or polishing cloth, and a lint-free cloth for glass

disinfectant liquid

dustpan and brush

furniture polish and/or oil

cream cleanser or scouring liquid

powder cleanser

glass cleaner

old toothbrush to clean hard-to-get-at nooks and crannies

rubber gloves

scouring pads

scrubbing brush

sponge mop

sponges

vacuum cleaner bags

 PUT A BRUSH AND HOLDER BEHIND EACH LOO. This means you never have to move one around and it encourages others to clean the toilet more often.

Rationalise recipes

We've all got a tottering pile or a messy folder packed with random clippings and notes that constitute a recipe collection. Sometimes it's something you've seen in a magazine that you've pulled out and put away to make one day; or it might be Great-Auntie Kath's famous recipe for lemon delicious, in her spidery, faded handwriting. The alternative to this clutter is simple and quick:

Buy a big ringbinder with plastic sheet protectors Twenty-five sheet protectors is a good working number.

Install divider tabs Then write categories on them, such as 'Chicken', 'Soup', 'Fish', 'Mincemeat', 'Desserts', 'Pasta', and so on.

Trim all your clippings Then slide them into the appropriate plastic sheet.

There are two big advantages to this system: one is that when you turn to the appropriate section, you will probably find you already had a recipe for butter chicken or similar. If the new recipe you've clipped has a more interesting twist, just toss the old one, and replace it with the new one. You can also create your own categories, such as 'Cheap', 'Fussy Eaters', 'Vegetarian', or 'Dinner for One'.

FOCUS ON UFOs. These are the Unfinished Objects that everyone has: half-knitted jumpers, half-stitched samplers, half-filled photo albums and so on. Pick one and stick at it for just 30 minutes every day until it's done. A short burst of concentrated effort is worth more than several hours with interruptions.

Review your wardrobe

If you can't open your wardrobe door without something falling on you from a top shelf, it's time to clean it out. By creating roomy hanging space, you will also avoid crushing your clothes and having to re-iron them. Here's how to get started:

Keep your wardrobe just for clothes Haul out the sewing box, Christmas wrapping paper, photo albums and tennis racquet. If you can't find homes or uses for these objects, put them in a box for charity.

Divide your wardrobe into three Allocate one half for long items, like dresses and coats, a second for shirts hanging on one pole, and then skirts and trousers hanging on a second pole underneath. Your local hardware store will have a list of local handymen who can install brackets if you can't do it yourself.

Group like items Hang shirts, trousers and jeans all together. Store out-of-season and rarely worn clothes, like evening wear, separately in moth-proof bags in the least accessible part of the wardrobe. Store related items next to each other where possible, for example, put socks right next to shoes.

Put hangers all in the same direction Toss out rusty or broken hangers, or recycle them.

Fold woollens carefully Keep them in moth-proof drawers or stackable, clear acrylic boxes in your wardrobe. Toss in a couple of moth-repellent sachets.

Organise all the smaller items Underwear, socks, belts, ties, beach gear and sport accessories should all go into either drawers or other storage holders, such as small plastic baskets or on specially designed hangers.

Keep shoes on a shoe rack You can also keep them in shoe bags hanging on the inside of the wardrobe door.

Iron things before you put them away Same goes for minor repairs, like sewing on buttons – do it before you put them away.

Rotate your summer and winter clothes Store whichever group is out of season in a second, secure, moth-proof wardrobe. If you haven't got the space, invest in plastic hanging wardrobes or bags.

 DON'T HANG JUMPERS OR KNITWEAR. They will develop sad, droopy shoulders and strange, uneven hemlines.

Let go of clothes

Take your life in your own hands, and what happens?
A terrible thing – no one else to blame.

ERICA JONG, AUTHOR

Most of us have clothes in our wardrobe we will never wear again. These items can clutter the space and, even though it's sometimes hard to get rid of them, it's an important thing to do. Here's how:

Take the two-year test The usual rule is that if you haven't worn it in two years you should get rid of it. This doesn't always apply, depending on what you have – classic shirts and skirts, for example, should last for several years. Also, sentimental items are exempt: a wedding dress may be kept, but the magenta dyed-to-match bridesmaid's shoes may not.

Try on everything you intend to keep This can be disheartening, but if you don't like what you see in the mirror when you put that skirt on, why keep looking at it hanging in the wardrobe?

✳ BUY CLASSIC CLOTHES. Carefully chosen well-cut items that don't date will reduce the amount of clothes you have to throw away.

Fix up your photos

Have you got drawers or shoe boxes full of old photos? Here's how to reduce them to a number and format people can look at and enjoy – not to mention reclaim all the space they're taking up:

Round them all up Check the house thoroughly – there are bound to be several storage places.

Sort into chronological order If you're lucky, the processing date will be on the packet or the photos themselves. Put strays that don't seem to fit in anywhere to one side until you've finished checking all the packets. Hopefully, your memory will be jogged and you'll find where they belong. If creating a full chronology is just too daunting, consider grouping photos in another way: by occasion (Christmas, birthday celebration, wedding), by year (a broad category, but at least imposes some sort of order) or by trip. You might want to add a date, for example, 'Africa 1990' or 'Christmas 1979'.

Weed ruthlessly! Like most people, you will have occasional gems interspersed among a much larger collection of very ordinary photos, plus duplicates. Starting with the oldest photos, go through the pile one at a time. Ask yourself, 'Do I want to see this again?' 'Will other people?' Cull all the shots that are overexposed, underexposed or blurred. If it passes these tests, it's a keeper; if not, toss it. Try to make the editorial decision rapidly, otherwise you'll weaken. Don't do this job when your children are around, otherwise they're bound to want to look at the photos with you. The ultimate aim is to keep all the best photos for yourself, with the others being shared out to family and friends. If you've got children, it's a nice idea to make them an album out of the photographs you don't keep.

Don't be negative If you want to keep the negs, place them in envelopes with the date and a brief description on the outside. Attach the envelopes to the inside of the album where the pictures are displayed, or file them in the back of the appropriate photo storage box.

IDENTIFY PHOTOS. Before you arrange your photos in albums or file them in boxes, write the names of the subjects, the location and the approximate date on the back. We all have old family photos that no one can identify with any certainty. The next generation to enjoy this wonderful collection you've made will bless you for doing it. Same goes for slides, home movies or videotapes.

Remember dates

In France, women have the right to age. Everywhere else, it seems women must be perfect, or they are judged a failure.

CATHERINE DENEUVE

Here's how to remember all the personal dates that are important to you:

Make a master list of names Include all of the important people in your life – friends, family and work associates. For everyone on this list, find out birthdays and other important anniversary dates, and enter this information next to their names. File this master list in your filing cabinet under 'Personal' or something similar, and review and update it at the beginning of each year.

Note dates in your diary and calendar Write all birthday or anniversary information on the relevant day in red.

Use personal organiser software It will save you from carrying around a diary and/or address book. You type in notes and information with a stylus. You can also enter all important dates and lists, and then reminders will pop up automatically. Some have Internet connection so you can view and edit documents, videos, photos and browse Web contents offline.

Send yourself a reminder Some office software packages will include an electronic diary. You can set it up so that you are automatically reminded of special dates.

 DON'T FORGET BIRTHDAYS. Sending a card or email or making a phone call to someone on their birthday can remind that person how important they are to you.

Planning essentials
The containers

Choosing the right sort of storage containers is the first step towards tidying up, especially if your home has insufficient cupboards and wardrobes. Here are some of my favourites:

Stackable drawer sets Discount stores such as Ikea and Freedom regularly turn out a new series of these, usually in inexpensive plywood or a printed cardboard cut-out that you fold into shape yourself. They are terrific for all sorts of small, loose items, e.g. stationery, Lego, small toys and sewing requirements.

Tool boxes Sturdy, lightweight plastic tool or fishing tackle boxes with one or two divided shelves are marvellous for organising hobby and game materials.

CD racks There is a wide variety of different types, from mini desktop towers to ones that stand on the floor next to the sound system. However, for the sake of neatness and to maintain the quality of your CDs, it's best to keep them in lidded containers away from dust.

Trollies on wheels These are best for storing heavier items that you don't want to be hauling out of cupboards, e.g. shoes, bags and toys, cooking equipment and garden tools. Some varieties come with removable shelves and CD racks that slot in one on top of the other.

Mesh baskets Use these in the kitchen, either under the kitchen sink or on the benchtop, for collecting together and storing cleaning items. Choose pretty plastic, wire or woven ones for the bathroom to hold face washers, soaps, cottonballs, buds or wool, and bottles. Larger plastic baskets or trays are good for organising clothes-washing products.

Wire stacking drawers These are a great idea for getting more mileage out of wardrobes or cupboards that haven't been fitted with shelving, especially if you're renting and so not in a position to permanently modify the existing storage. Look for models with adjustable-depth drawers, so that you can vary items you keep in them.

A lockable metal cabinet This is a must for medical supplies if you have small children.

The catalogues

Every week there are handfuls of catalogues stuffed into the letterbox, and it's tempting to just put them straight into the recycle bin. However, they can sometimes be a useful resource. Here's how:

Put them aside Get into the habit of putting them to one side when you check your mail.

Flip through them At a regular time every day or so – perhaps as you're eating breakfast, or stacking the dishwasher at night – quickly flip through them and tag or tear out anything of interest.

Keep an eye out for supermarket and pharmacy specials This is especially important as Christmas approaches. They're excellent for giving you ideas about different things to buy, and you can save a lot of money by purchasing the reduced items ahead of time. Same goes for toys and garden equipment. These catalogues often contain coupons that entitle you to a discount on a specified item if you take it to the shop within a certain time frame.

Regularly throw things out Throw away and recycle any clippings or catalogues you don't need or that have gone past their buy-by date.

From birth to age 18, a girl needs good parents.
From 18 to 35, she needs good looks.
From 35 to 45, she needs a good personality.
From 45 on, she needs good cash.

SOPHIE TUCKER, RUSSIAN-BORN BLUES SINGER

Win the money war

Face financial facts

Your finances require constant attention so you can stay ahead, and not get caught out by unexpected bills and market changes, such as interest rate hikes, or changes to bank fees. These routines help you take charge of your money and keep things flowing smoothly:

Track your cash If you can't work out where all your hard-earned cash is going, write down everything you spend for a month, from your morning cup of coffee, to kids' pocket money, to your train ticket home, so you can see exactly what happens to it. Then work out where you can save money. Easy ways to cut daily expenditure include eating breakfast at home, making your own lunch and, if possible, walking or cycling to work. Use the money you've saved to pay off debts such as credit card bills, beginning with the ones with the highest interest rates. If you don't have any debts, start a savings plan and set up a monthly amount to pay into it.

Set up direct debits and use B-pay Do this for as many bills as possible, including council rates, utilities, credit cards, cable TV and tolls. That way you won't get big, unexpected bills, and you won't have to remember to pay them.

Bank via the Internet, rather than waste time in queues In addition to having access to your financial information 24 hours a day, 7 days a week, you'll be able to check loan details, find out how much interest you've earned and transfer funds.

Be prepared Keep all other bills in a display folder with clear plastic pages inside. When a bill comes, highlight the amount and the due date. Place the bill in the folder, in order of due date. Always check the small print – an insurance renewal, for example, may request 25 May as the due date for payment, but on reading the terms and conditions, you will probably find that you have a period of 30 days grace. The bill that needs to be paid first should be at the front of the folder. This way you can see at a glance the companies you owe money to and when they have to be paid.

USE THE PHONE OR INTERNET TO PAY BILLS. It takes only a few minutes to set up your accounts – water, gas, electricity, phone and credit cards, for example – and you'll save on postage, as well as time.

Go shopping for a bank

A bank is a place that will only lend you money if you can prove that you don't need it.

BOB HOPE, ACTOR AND COMEDIAN

Choosing a bank is like shopping for most things – firstly you need to decide on the features that are most important to you, then you need to start comparing the different services on offer. Pick up all the relevant brochures and forms from a short list of, say, three banks, then sit down and read the small print. These are the main areas where things can come unstuck:

Minimum balance requirements Many styles of accounts have a high minimum balance you need to maintain to avoid paying additional fees and to earn interest. If you expect a lot of movement in your account, you do not want to have to pay for the privilege of the bank holding your money.

Interest payments Just because one bank offers a higher rate of interest doesn't mean you're going to be any better off. You will get a much more representative view if you compare the different banks' methods of calculating that interest. The best option is to receive compound interest on your daily balance. This means you earn interest – including the previously accumulated interest – every day. Avoid accounts that only pay interest on your balance after your deposits have cleared, or which only pay interest on your lowest balance during any set time frame, such as a month.

Service charges Costs for ATM transactions and bank fees can vary widely, from being free to costing between $1 and $10 per transaction.

Cheque accounts Choose an account that offers 10 to 15 free cheques a month as opposed to one that charges for every cheque, irrespective of the number used.

 MAKE BANKS EARN YOUR BUSINESS. Visit the bank manager in person. Ask for a detailed list of charges you might have to pay with your proposed new account. Ask about ways *they* can save *you* money: for example, will they reduce fees and charges if you have more than one account, or if you take out a loan with them? Ask if you can reduce monthly service charges if you bank exclusively online.

Find a good accountant

The tax laws are so complex today it's a mistake not to hire a professional. Yes, they charge – but they can do in a day what might take you a week. Relying on a financial professional not only makes your day-to-day work easier because you can concentrate on what you are good at, but it can make all the difference to long-term financial progress. Here are the key questions to ask:

How do they structure their fees? Most accountancy businesses have different levels of staff, from senior to junior. However, the work they do may be charged to you at different rates, or they may work on a flat-fee basis, regardless of how many hours are involved or who does the work. Call the Society of Australian Certified Practising Accountants and get an estimate of what you might expect to pay for financial planning advice and/or preparation of returns, so that you have a guide.

Do they charge for occasional advice? Some firms charge like wounded bulls if you ask even one simple question over the phone. Others may regard a small query as part of the ongoing relationship.

Who are their clients? Ask about their background. Some companies gear their practice towards particular professions, or small businesses, for example. How long have they been in practice? Do they have any special services that, ideally, match your needs? Check they are registered. As a general rule, pick someone who has at least 10 years experience rather than someone who's new.

Are they tied to any particular financial service? Avoid any accountant or financial planner who has strong ties to any one bank, stockbroking house, insurance agency or superannuation fund. Walk away even faster if they have a financial affiliation, as they probably earn commission on any services they manage to sell you. Unfortunately, many financial planners are not much better than insurance agents or stockbrokers looking for sales so it's far better to go with someone who makes their money on a fee-only basis. If you are looking for investment advice, ask them what sources of information they use and why.

 ASK FOR REFERENCES. Ask the referee how the accountant has worked out for them, and what they've done. Don't even consider someone who won't give you names of current clients.

*I've been rich and I've been poor.
Rich is better.*

SOPHIE TUCKER

Demystify tax

You may be storing decades worth of cheque butts, receipts and bits and pieces of paper because of a morbid fear of the tax office. Like many of us, you're convinced you'll need all of these records forever, just in case there's ever a problem with an audit. These are the basic rules to follow:

Keep proof of your sources of income For most people, that's going to mean a tax declaration form and a group certificate from your employer. If you're self-employed or run a small business, it's going to involve keeping copies of all your quarterly Business Activity Statements and payments, as well as your annual tax return. Same goes for self-funded retirees, who derive their income from managed funds, investments or other sources, such as rental properties. Save all the relevant pieces of paper, plus all the receipts and paperwork that substantiate any deductions you may have made, e.g. charitable contributions, medical benefits funds, and other business-related expenses.

Organise your tax records by financial year Depending on how much paperwork is involved, you'll need a document box for each year. Put all papers related to income and deductions for this year into the box. Label it, 'Tax, (2002-3)'. As you go through the financial year, pop any receipts straight into an envelope in the top of the box, labelled 'Receipts'. Every quarter, sort these loose receipts into groups, e.g. 'Stationery', 'Couriers/Taxis/Fares', 'Telephone', 'Newspapers and Magazines', and so on.

Write cheque numbers on receipts If you use your cheque account for expenses that you will be claiming as tax deductions, get into the habit of writing the cheque number on the receipts you put in your 'Tax' file. Keep old cheque butts for the term of the current tax year.

Keep a separate file or box labelled 'Home' Keep in this file or box all the papers that contain basic information about your property, such as the title or rental agreement, council maps, pest inspection certificates and repairs. If you are claiming a percentage of the mortgage or rental as a tax deduction, you will need to keep duplicates of bank statements in your 'Tax' file as well.

 KEEP BUSINESS AND PERSONAL RECORDS SEPARATE. If you work from home, try to have a credit card, cheque account and telephone line devoted exclusively to your business activities. If this isn't possible, and you use some items, such as your car, phone or computer, for both purposes, faithfully keep a log of these expenses.

Deduct and prosper

Even if you have enlisted the services of a savvy accountant, it's easy to overlook tax deductions that you are entitled to claim. Here are some thought-starters – check with your accountant to see if any are appropriate to you:

Books and magazines This can cover both those reading materials directly relevant to your sphere of business as well as any books, magazines, newspapers or newsletters related to tax or finance – your daily newspaper, for example.

Charitable out-of-pocket expenses If you have donated your personal time to a tax-deductible charitable organisation, you might be able to claim related expenses, e.g. petrol, parking, meters and tolls. So if, for example, you regularly speak to community groups, or spend an afternoon a month helping a local charity, this can add up to quite a substantial amount of petty cash outlay.

Health insurance The rules vary from fund to fund and even from state to state in Australia, but, if you are self-employed, it is worth investigating to see if you are able to deduct all or some of the premium you pay for your own insurance. Same goes for personal or life insurance, and possibly home and contents insurance, if you work from home.

Miscellaneous business expenses Even if you are a PAYE employee you may find that some of your business expenses not reimbursed by your employer may be deductible. For example, use of your car, or cost of public transport or taxis for business purposes; business use of a mobile phone which you own, or of pay phones for business purposes; stationery, office supplies and photocopying; self-education (e.g. courses and seminars, including all or part of costs of travel, accommodation and food); gifts to business associates and clients; costs involved in decorating office premises, either your employer's or your home-based workplace (e.g. lamps, fresh flowers); and, in some cases, entertainment for business purposes.

 KEEP TRACK OF MONEY you spend on your home. The amount you spend on things like renovations, plumbing and rewiring won't be deductible on your annual income tax, but it may reduce the taxable gain when your house is sold in years to come.

Get the most from your insurance

If you own your own home, you must have an insurance policy that covers you against damage to the property, and loss or theft of the contents. Ideally, the policy should also protect against injury to anyone on your property. Here's a check list of what to look for when shopping around for a policy that suits you:

Go for more, not less Most experts recommend that the amount your property is insured for represents around 80 per cent of your home's value. However, it's important that you ask a professional property appraiser or real estate agent, whose judgment you trust, for an idea of what this figure might be – most people drastically undervalue their home and contents, and they are surprised to learn what their assets are actually worth.

Take a long, hard look Home and personal insurance policies don't come cheaply, so research it thoroughly. Most will cover major risks, such as fire and theft. Some may offer cover for earthquakes, drought or flood as optional extras – if you think this is a potential problem, it's worth paying the extra.

Be clear on what you're getting When reading the fine print, be aware of the difference between being paid the actual value of lost or damaged goods (you receive the replacement cost of your item, minus the value of its depreciation) and the replacement value (you should be able to replace the item at today's prices). Naturally, a policy which offers replacement value on all or major items is going to be more expensive than one which offers actual value, but you may still end up ahead when you take into account what you're really getting.

Ask about special cover All companies will have an optional program that covers rare or irreplaceable items, e.g. jewellery, stamps, antiques, maps, art. You may need to organise an independent assessment of the items in question, and pay for certificates of authentication.

 REDUCE YOUR FEES. All insurance companies will bring their prices down on a sliding scale if you comply with certain requirements, such as installing deadlocks, security screens and doors, or sensor lights. And using one insurance company for all your needs, if you can, should make you eligible for discounts and lower premiums.

*Money can't buy you happiness –
but it does bring you a more pleasant
form of misery.*

SPIKE MILLIGAN

Buying a car

To avoid being taken for a ride (and I don't mean a test drive) do your homework first. To buy the car you want at the lowest possible price, follow these steps:

Consider the car you've got now How much is it worth? Get a professional valuation, and then decide whether you want to sell it yourself or trade it in on your new car.

Do the numbers Work out how much money you can comfortably afford to repay each month. Many car dealerships offer enticing deals with tiny up-front deposits. However, you're going to be much better off financially if you can put as much towards your initial deposit as possible, as this will then lower your monthly repayments. If you are leasing the car with the aim of running it as a tax loss against business expenses, ask your accountant to work out an optimum lease repayment figure.

Consider second hand cars If you are buying a second-hand car, take a car-savvy friend with you to check it out. Always arrange for an independent vehicle inspection from an appropriate organisation in your state, such as the NRMA, or the RACV. Avoid paying in cash, and never leave without a receipt and all the relevant documents, warranties and manuals.

Look at lots of different cars Just because your best friend has a certain make of car, doesn't mean it will suit your needs. Go to dealerships and ask for test drives of new and second-hand cars, and make it crystal clear you're only there to look, not buy.

Shop around for a loan You may be in a position to combine your new car loan with your home mortgage loan, or to roll it into a business overdraft. Remember to factor in your on-road costs, such as insurance and registration fees. Car salesmen are notorious for forgetting to mention these until you're committed to what you think is a final price.

 BE ON YOUR GUARD. There haven't been all those jokes about car salesmen over the years for no reason. Always go to a reputable dealer who is accredited with the Motor Traders' Association of Australia. If buying privately, always arrange for independent vehicle inspections.

… and looking after it

A woman's rule of thumb: if it has tyres or testicles,
you're going to have trouble with it.

GRAFFITI

Cars are not, generally speaking, something that women spend much time thinking about. However, ignorance is not bliss when it comes to owning and running one. The better you take care of it, the better it will take care of you. Here's what you need to do:

Familiarise yourself with the manual Different cars require different service routines and maintenance at different times. Being savvy about your car's particular requirements will reduce the likelihood of your paying for unnecessary services from unscrupulous technicians.

Check the basics regularly Oil and drive belts should be checked approximately every 5000 kilometres. Check water and other fluids (brake, battery, transmission and airconditioner coolant) regularly, and especially before you go on a long trip. Check tyre pressure at least once a month and get into the habit of looking for scratches or signs of wear. Check your lights regularly, front and back. Same goes for windscreen wipers – use your windscreen water jets to see how well they are working, even if it's not raining. Top up the windscreen water reservoir regularly. And check your spare tyre every couple of months to make sure it hasn't gone down.

Have a safety inspection Some Australian states require an annual safety inspection in order to renew car registration. Even if you have a new car or it's not legally necessary, get it done anyway.

Keep a service record Keep a record of the receipts from having your car serviced, noting the date and the mileage. When you want to sell your car or trade it in, you'll have a tangible service record which may get you a higher price.

 PACK A ROADSIDE EMERGENCY KIT and keep it in the car at all times. It should contain a copy of your insurance and registration papers; a warning device, such as a flare or reflective triangle; jumper cables; a first aid kit; a flashlight with extra batteries; a plastic container of water; and a fire-extinguisher.

Save on car insurance

Never lend your car to anyone to whom you have given birth.

ERMA BOMBECK, COMEDIENNE

One of the biggest expenses associated with running a car is keeping up with the payment of the insurance premiums, especially as the car gets older. Here are some tips on getting the best – and lowest – possible policy:

Shop around Just like home and personal insurance, doing your homework and comparing deals can save you a lot of money. Premiums have been known to vary by more than 30 per cent between different insurance companies.

Pool your resources It pays to put your eggs in one basket and use one company for several policies. It's also worth asking if they offer an additional discount if you are insuring more than one car for the same household or business.

Steer clear of flash cars The higher the profile of the car you drive, the more you're going to pay to drive it. Luxury cars cost more to fix and replace, so insurance companies have a different, higher fee structure for them.

Install safety features For example, getting a car alarm should lower your premium.

 TRADE ON YOUR RECORD. Having an accident-free record should score you a lower rate. If the insurer doesn't mention it, ask. Some companies also offer lower premiums for drivers who have done defensive-driving classes.

Shop, but don't drop

I love clothes but, for the most part, I find shopping for them a disheartening and expensive experience. Unless you're a diehard shopping junkie, try these tips:

Only upgrade twice a year Review and, if necessary, replace some of your clothes to coincide with the beginning of summer and winter. Work out exactly what you need to buy. A good idea is to purchase just one complete smart-casual outfit – say, a trouser suit and shirt, or a dress and jacket ensemble, plus shoes and bag – every season. In less than two years you'll have half-a-dozen terrific outfits you can always rely on to make you look and feel good.

Plan a biannual list for the major sales These usually boast substantial savings so your list should include necessities such as bras, pantyhose, shirts and jeans. Keep a list of your children's current clothing sizes in your wallet. If you see the perfect gift idea or a bargain at the sales, you can take advantage of your discovery then and there.

Buy drip-dry This cuts down on items that require ironing or drycleaning.

Investigate the Internet There is a huge range of shopping options, especially for items that don't really need to be tried on, such as plain T-shirts, sleepwear, men's and kids' clothes and underwear. Many sites have weekly and monthly specials that are often substantially cheaper than regular shops.

 BUY QUALITY. The better the quality of the clothes, the less time and effort involved in maintaining them.

Crafty shopping strategies

In every home there will always be the emergency dash to the local corner store for milk and bread. However, shopping this way on a regular basis is a huge time-waster, not to mention expensive. Organising food for a household is just one of those jobs that has to be done. These ideas make it easier.

Set up accounts with your local butcher, baker and greengrocer Place an order by telephone every week, asking for it to be delivered at a time when you'll be there. If you open charge accounts, the store will often notify you of special sales and discounts.

Shop on the Internet Major supermarkets now have online ordering facilities. There are also many highly professional, cost-effective suppliers of food; www.aussiegrocer.com.au and www.shopfast.com.au are just two of them.

Shop at less busy times Going first thing on a Sunday morning or on a weeknight means shorter queues.

Buy in bulk You can make terrific savings at warehouses and markets on everyday commodities such as meat, bread, pet food, paper products and toiletries. Shop every three months, and load up. You should especially double up on non-perishable items you use often and run out of quickly.

Use mail-order catalogues They enable you to shop whenever you like, for example, while you're waiting for an appointment, or in the evening in front of TV.

Shop for food only once a week The secret is always taking a list, to avoid both the frustration of forgotten items and the unnecessary expense of buying something you don't really need. Keep the list handy in the kitchen and write items down as soon as you think of them.

Go shopping on a full stomach You'll buy less food on impulse.

Combine errands When you go to the supermarket, do other things while you're out and about, such as dropping off the drycleaning or picking up a prescription. Even though it takes longer, it will take four times as long to make the trips separately.

 CARRY A CALCULATOR. They don't take up much more room than a credit card, and are very handy for dividing a bill or comparing prices.

Buying a major appliance

It is only when they go wrong that machines remind you how powerful they are.

CLIVE JAMES, AUSTRALIAN CRITIC

Purchasing a fridge, drier, washing machine, dishwasher, freezer or stove is a major investment that pays considerable dividends by helping to save you time and effort, so you can enjoy home life more. Here's what to look for:

Identify features that are important to you For example, if you have allergies, get a vacuum cleaner with a Hepa filter. Ask friends with similar appliances for their opinions.

Factor in store extras A higher-priced fridge that comes with free delivery may work out cheaper than another with a hefty delivery fee, for example.

Try for a trade-in You are often able to get credit on an older model.

Shop locally It can save you time and money, as smaller stores need to make themselves as attractive to you as possible compared with the national chains.

Insist on seeing the product in action Otherwise you won't really know if it's easy to use, or if it's too noisy, and so on.

Complete the warranty card straightaway File the owner portion with the sales receipt. If something breaks down, you can quickly work out how to get it serviced or replaced.

 STUDY THE WARRANTY before you buy the item so you know what the manufacturer promises to cover and for how long.

Planning essentials
The calculator

Most of us use a calculator every day, but this doesn't necessarily mean we're using it to our best advantage. A calculator can help you decide what to do and what to ask, especially when shopping or working out your finances. Here's how to make sure yours is working for you:

Assess your needs How will you be using your calculator? Just for totting up household accounts at tax time? Or for more complicated study or work-related uses? You may only require a slim, inexpensive credit card-sized one to slip in your wallet or Filofax, or you may get more use from a larger desk model with a memory and printable adding facility.

Do your homework Familiarise yourself with what's available at home electronics stores. Prices vary considerably, depending on features offered, which you may or may not require.

Buy a reputable one Stick with a name you know. A 'home' brand or cheap model from a discount store might be less expensive, but you could find it's a false economy should it start to malfunction.

Check bills and bank statements Keep on top of your finances by double-checking amounts and by balancing your cheque book. It's surprising how often institutions make mistakes!

Compare costs Take a calculator with you when grocery shopping; it's a handy way of comparing costs per serving. Do a quick currency conversion if making a purchase over the Internet.

The Internet

Begin the process of choosing a financial planner, an accountant or an investment opportunity such as stock trading by first doing an Internet search. Are you looking for information about cash management and budgeting? Or trying to choose a retirement plan or make other investments? Or are you doing tax and estate planning, investigating your insurance needs or reviewing your financial goals? The Internet is the place to start researching all aspects of your financial needs, and many institutions offer special introductory deals that are worth pursuing. Here are the questions to ask:

What are their professional credentials? Most Internet-based companies are happy to provide evidence of standards of business practice, memberships, client history, and so on. Naturally, if they do not, steer clear.

How long have they been in business? Your money and your future are on the line. Don't put them in the hands of any company who's new to the business. Look for companies with at least 10 years experience; this increases the likelihood that you'll be working with professionals.

What is their investment philosophy? Certain investment companies lean more towards different types of investments, such as mutual funds, futures trading, real estate, blue-chip stocks etc.

Ask for references Before you commit to a financial plan or take up an option, ask for the names and numbers of clients the company has worked with for at least three years. Call them and ask whether their experiences have lived up to their expectations.

Trade online This is an increasingly popular way to trade stocks and may well become the main way to execute such transactions in the future. The advantage to you? It's less expensive and more flexible than standard trading options.

I'll tell you what is the best of all life has to offer – to be able to howl with laughter with a friend because you think the same things are funny.

GLORIA VANDERBILT

Let the good times roll

Laughter: the best medicine

My mother always used to say, 'If I didn't laugh, I'd cry'. Still, old habits are hard to break – when we're taught to be 'good girls', we're also told to 'stop being silly'. Now that we're bigger, being serious makes us feel intelligent and in control. But the simplest chuckle can be enough to break the stress cycle. My favourite ways to get through the days also stop me from taking myself too seriously:

Scream and shout The next time pressure mounts, just imagine yourself whooping at the top of your voice and it will lighten your mood. Better yet, open your mouth and shout, 'Enough, already!'

Be a drama queen Dredge a laugh out of a last-straw-breaking-the-camel's-back type of situation by exaggerating your reaction to it. Someone's left wet towels on the bathroom floor again? Fling your wrist to your forehead and go for it: 'MY GOD! Not again! I can't stand it! In fact – I feel faint. I have to lie down.'

Have a laugh fest Rent some comedy classics (*Annie Hall* and *The Blues Brothers* do it for me every time). Pore over comics, or read light-hearted, witty stories.

Spin out If you can't step backwards from stress mentally, do it physically. Stand up from your desk, say whatever's bugging you out loud, and then spin around in circles. It's a liberating thing to do, and gives some distance between you and the problem.

Play The next time you're feeling anxious or stressed, take a break and do something childish. Find crayons and draw a picture, blow bubbles, play with a yo-yo or play with some of your favourite old toys and games.

 FORCE A SMILE. Dr Bernie Siegel, an expert in the field of mind-body medicine, has said that even if you just pretend to be happy, by forcing a smile or a laugh, your body will still react by producing less of the stress hormone cortisol.

Girl talk

It's the friends you can call up at 4 am that matter.

MARLENE DIETRICH, GERMAN FILM STAR

Most women say their friendships with other women are among the most significant in their lives. This becomes even more true the older you get, as you realise these relationships are an investment in the future. Sure, your family knows you too, but with them you play a certain role – you're looked at in a certain way. Female friends allow you to be yourself. Here's how to keep existing friendships strong, and develop good quality new ones:

Run away together Invite friends on retreats to a health farm, fishing, a country vineyard or a road trip to somewhere you've all wanted to go.

Eat out Not much beats talking over dinner with the girls. Women's tendency to 'tend and befriend', to seek comfort and to support each other, helps explain why they live an average of seven and a half years longer than men. Stress has a way of dissipating when women surround themselves with women.

Be mindful of negative emotions Issues involving envy and competition are damaging to women's friendships. Recognise those feelings and try to handle them openly.

Share your feelings It's important not only to listen to and support your friends, but also to confide your thoughts and experiences with them. When someone opens up to you, it's a gift. It says, 'I trust you'.

Be there When my father died and I was going through a divorce, a girlfriend came over on my birthday, got me into my pyjamas, brushed my hair, and tucked me up on the couch in front of a funny video while she put the boys to bed, folded the laundry, and ironed the school shirts. It was one of the most life-affirming and selfless acts I have experienced.

Expand your circle A good first step is to think of someone you know casually – at work or a neighbour – and ask her out for coffee. Book clubs can also be great friendship builders.

 TELL FRIENDS HOW YOU FEEL. Just saying, 'You're so important to me' or, 'I really value our relationship', can strengthen a friendship.

Bring back that sexual spark

Sex is extremely good for you. As well as feeling great, it helps reduce stress and can boost your relationship. But the pressures of modern living can make the best sex life dull and monotonous. If you feel that you could do the whole thing in your sleep because it's all so familiar, here's how to spice things up a little:

Talk to each other Going off sex is very often triggered by some other issue in the relationship. Talking openly about problems reduces the chances of bottling up other resentments.

Figure out what you want It might take some courage if you're not in the habit of pushing boundaries, but a tender, curious approach and experimentation can be very arousing. You don't have to be outrageous at all – just revealing your desires or having fun helps get you out of the rut of a sex life that's become just a habit. Shake things up a bit, change your routine and use your imagination.

Choose your time Don't have sex when you're tired or sick, or just for the sake of it, or to make the other person happy. All of these motives will backfire on both of you. Interestingly, our body clocks are generally more primed for sex first thing in the morning – another good incentive for waking up a little earlier.

Take it slowly In our race to get everything done, there's a temptation to skip the kissing and cuddling of foreplay. Don't just kiss on the lips either, kiss your partner's ears, wrists, neck, all sorts of nifty new pleasure spots. Turn the lights down or use only a soft lamp. Bright lights can be a big turn-off.

Enjoy a massage Relaxing with your partner will arouse sensual feelings. Massage each other, take a bath or spa together, watch a sexy movie, or go into a sex shop for inspiration.

Get fit for sex Surveys repeatedly show that fitness levels and body confidence are strongly linked with regular sex. Feeling comfortable with your physique is one of the first steps to being relaxed about sex. As well as working on overall fitness, work specifically to strengthen your pelvic floor muscles (found around the vaginal area and used to control your flow of urine). All together now, squ-e-e-e-eze!

 PLAN AHEAD. It's not unromantic to book each other in for some time alone – ideally a weekend or at least a night away.

*As you go through life, you will
come to great chasms. Jump!
They are not as wide as you think.*

NATIVE AMERICAN SAYING

Have a good weekend

The really important thing about a weekend is that it should provide a change from what you do Monday to Friday. Even if it's busy, you can still feel refreshed at the end of it if you have done something different, no matter how small. I like to make a slow-cooking soup or a casserole, then do a jigsaw puzzle with my kids – two things I find very effective in putting work-related thoughts right out of my mind. Your weekend should be a reward. Here are some ideas to factor in some fun:

Set aside some time for something quite different For example, exploring an antique warehouse, going to the aquarium or model train display – anything that presents a complete change from what you do during the week. Sticking to a relatively short time span, say an hour or two, makes it more likely you can manage the extra activity without missing out on other commitments.

Prune weekend chores to a minimum If new seedlings have to be put in, then do it – but set yourself a time to finish the job and stick to it. Give yourself a reward afterwards, for example, go out for coffee.

Plan an overnight holiday for at least one weekend a year It doesn't have to be expensive. My friend Suzanne booked an inexpensive city hotel room and took her kids sightseeing for two days, visiting parks, taking photos and enjoying buskers and other free street entertainment.

 CREATE SPACE FOR TEENAGERS. Encourage teenagers to bring their friends home on the weekend by providing plenty of food and a relatively private space. It helps if you have a liberal attitude towards mess. Remember that it saves you having to ferry them around as much.

Plan the perfect party

When you're busy, it's always the pleasurable aspects of life – like having people over for a meal or a celebration – that get put on the back burner. However, with just a little bit of thinking ahead, you don't have to get stressed about it. Here's how:

Make two lists A shopping list of everything you need to buy, and a task list of all the things you'd like to get done before the party.

Write your guest list at least three weeks before the party The invitation – whether written, emailed or phoned through – should let your guests know whether dinner will be served. Unless you're going formal or fancy dress, a dress code is probably not necessary.

Plan ahead Make sure you plan the menu, or call a caterer, two weeks ahead of time. If you're hiring linen, glasses, plates and cutlery, order them two weeks ahead, and pick it all up (or have it delivered) the day before. Same goes for extra chairs and trestle tables.

Get help If you're inviting more than ten people, give serious thought to hiring an extra pair of hands to take coats, serve drinks and hand around food. Explain exactly what you want the helper to do. If it's a large teenage party, security guards are an unfortunate necessity in these times.

Buy drinks and mixers well ahead of time If it's a large order, ask your bottle shop to deliver the booze chilled, on the day. Don't forget plenty of non alcoholic drinks. Arrange for someone to collect ice on the morning of the party and stash it wherever you're planning to keep bottles and cans.

Prevent breakages Clear away any unnecessary clutter and family paraphernalia – if it's not in the way, it won't get knocked over or broken.

Make sure the bathroom is clean Put out nice soaps and clean handtowels. Put out extra toilet paper, too.

Give some thought to music Select some CDs, and, unless you're having a dance party, keep the music at a low enough level that guests can talk comfortably.

Put a drink in your hand Enjoy yourself!

 USE QUICK TRICKS. Fresh flowers and groups of candles can give a room an instant facelift and create a welcoming atmosphere in very little time.

Oh, God, my head

When you drink alcohol to excess, your body is unable to break it down fast enough, so it accumulates in a harmful by-product called acetyldehyde. The liver – which has the job of detoxifying your body – is overwhelmed by dealing with this substance, and that is what creates the awful feeling. The other main reason for a hangover is dehydration, because alcohol robs the body of water and, with this, vitamins and minerals. Here are some ways to combat hangovers:

Drink fruit juice It contains fructose, which helps the body burn alcohol faster. A large glass, in other words, will help accelerate removal of the alcohol still in your system the morning after.

Try toast and honey Honey is a very concentrated source of fructose, and eating a little the morning after is another way to help your body flush out whatever alcohol remains.

Drink bouillon Broth made from bouillon cubes or any homemade soup broth will help replace the salt and potassium your body loses when you drink.

Replenish your water supply Drinking plenty of water before you go to bed and again when you get up in the morning may help relieve discomfort caused by dehydration.

Take B-complex vitamins Research shows your system turns to B vitamins when it is under stress, and overtaxing your body with too much booze definitely qualifies as stress.

Get some pain relief A headache is invariably part of the package that goes with a hangover. Take aspirin or paracetamol.

Have something decent to eat If you can face it, that is. A balanced meal will replace the loss of essential nutrients. But keep the meal light: no fats or fried foods.

 LET TIME HEAL. The best and only foolproof cure for a hangover is, of course, 24 hours. Treat your symptoms as best you can. Get a good night's sleep and the next day – hopefully – all will be forgotten.

The real challenge in life is to always be looking forwards.

JOHN TRAVOLTA, ACTOR

Find holiday harmony

Too often, holidays (especially Christmas) are full of last-minute shopping expeditions and ringside seats to pointless annual sparring matches between relatives. It is possible, though, to mark the holidays in ways that help you reconnect to the things that really matter – family, community and faith. Here are some ideas to emphasise the spirit of togetherness:

Mend fences Focus on personal discovery and family ties. This is the time to ask Grandpa about his war experiences, and let him have the floor. Don't put it off.

Confront classic patterns Focus on the here and now. Your brother-in-law might try to whip up a political argument as he does every year – so change the subject to avoid hot spots.

Get help from friends Keep family functions non-confrontational by inviting a friend to tag along. Everyone will be on their best behaviour. Or, host a function for both friends and family.

Remember Put together a scrapbook of photos, stories or other memories of family occasions. Make it part of your holiday ritual to look through it every year and add to it.

Go for walks together There's something soothing about strolling, hand in hand. Breathe in, breathe out, and take stock: in the new year, how will you bring meaning to your life?

Don't try to please everyone In this age of blended families and long-distance relatives, it's impossible to please everyone. Instead, clearly communicate where you're going to spend festive meals ahead of time, decide how long you're going to stay, and don't compromise – if you only want to stay two hours at a certain get-together, stick to it.

CREATE NEW TRADITIONS. Just because people share your genes, doesn't mean they share your values. There are people who show up at every wedding and funeral, yet know nothing about anyone else. It's OK to put your happiness first and start traditions of your own. Spend the Easter weekend at a health retreat, or gather your own friends together for a Christmas Eve supper. The happiest holidays are the ones you celebrate with supportive people.

Keep kids entertained

If men had to have children, they would only ever have one each.

DIANA, PRINCESS OF WALES

Small, bored children, school holidays and a rainy day: a recipe for a screaming case of cabin fever? Or an opportunity to reconnect with the things that are really important, without having to spend money? These ideas can make the day a lot more fun for everyone:

Make something All you need are toothpicks, paper clips, paper, scissors, sticky tape and glue. You can make a fence, a house, a screen, a bridge, a farm, a tent . . . anything.

Cook something Always have an easy-to-make packet mix for muffins, biscuits or a cake on hand, preferably one that just needs to be stirred.

Play dress-ups Get out the box of old clothes that you have kept for school concert costume emergencies. Or haul out the charity bag with all the old clothes, caps, scarves and shoes that you're going to throw out anyway, and let your children do anything they want with them.

Get crafty Combine a little food colouring with water and a dash of rubbing alcohol, stir through dried pasta shapes briefly, then spread on newspapers to dry (the alcohol will make them dry much faster). String pasta for chains or necklaces, or paste different colours and shapes onto paper, to make a picture.

MAKE A CAMP. This was a great favourite with my boys. A large cardboard box can provide entertainment for hours. Failing that, they can mound up pillows and make a tent with rugs and blankets.

Make gift giving easier

*What would Christmas be without family? F**** excellent.*

CAR BUMPER STICKER

Do the words 'Christmas shopping' send your blood pressure skyrocketing? These tips will go a long way towards ensuring you save time, avoid stress, and still manage to come up with a gift that's just right:

Spend carefully That way you won't embarrass the recipient with an unexpectedly lavish present.

Make your list, then cross off as many as possible Buying fewer gifts will lower shopping stress considerably. Alternatives include drawing names out of a hat, so each person in the family only buys one gift for one other, or buying gifts only for children.

Start your Christmas shopping in July or August You'll save money as shopkeepers are notorious for jacking up prices in the lead-up to Christmas.

Shop when you're travelling or holidaying during the year Shopping while you're away is often more fun than when you're at home.

Give the same gift to several people on your list For example, sending a beautiful pot to each of your sisters, or giving homemade fudge to both sets of neighbours, is both thoughtful and efficient.

Shop online Many gift options are available quickly and easily via the Internet. Some fun and creative ideas include food (just about anything from gourmet gift baskets to scented teas), items from museum and art gallery shops (posters, cards, stationery, maps and all sorts of gizmos and novelties for kids) and gift certificates (massage, facial, pedicure). Steering clear of crowded department stores is the best way to keep your stress levels under control.

 CONSIDER PERSONAL TASTES. If you don't know someone that well, don't assume what they'd like by giving them a CD or book. A good bottle of wine is always a safe standby for, say, a business associate.

Recharge your relationships

Taking time to be a friend to yourself and to others should never be seen as time wasted, but rather as an investment in yourself. Here are some ideas for creating extra time for relationships:

Check your to-do list every day Swap one of the less important activities with something that will help build a relationship with a friend or family member. This could be a simple phone call, or dropping someone a quick email or letter. The critical thing is that you recognise this one relationship-enhancing effort as being just as important as all your other tasks and commitments.

Slow down Force yourself to reclaim your personal life. Schedule dates with your friends, partner or spouse. Call family members just to say a quick hello or to share an idea during the middle of the day. Plan social outings in advance and treat those commitments as seriously as you would a business meeting.

Create opportunities to be together When asked, most women will say their partner and/or children are the most important things in the world to them, and they want more time with them. Plan a regular Sunday night dinner, take a drive, do some shopping. It's during these informal encounters that some of the best conversations take place.

Make regular dates I have one group of girlfriends who all love to cook and entertain. We book a regular night every second month to go to each other's homes on a rotating basis, and each of us prepare something really delicious to eat. The trick is to book the date ahead, otherwise it won't happen.

 STOCK UP ON CARDS to say 'Thank you', 'Congratulations' and 'Well done'. Remember how you feel when a good word is sent your way, and be generous in your compliments to others – little kindnesses oil the wheels that make family, friend and work relationships go round.

Planning essentials
The food

Keep these tips about party food planning in mind as you get ready for any occasion:

Stick with classics If you want to try an ambitious new recipe, do it at a small dinner party, not if you're having a big 'do'. Generally speaking, simple favourites like cheese dips for hors d'oeuvres and a chicken casserole for a buffet are likely to appeal to a greater number of guests.

Work out quantities If you're planning a cocktail party, remember that guests will eat between four and six hors d'oeuvres in an hour and a half. So, for a three hour party with 20 people, you'll need between 160 and 240 pieces. Same goes for a party where you'll be serving lunch or supper – work out how many servings of rice, salad, meat or hot dishes each person is likely to have, then multiply it by the number of guests and work out quantities from there.

Mix it up Vary the flavours, textures and temperatures. If you have two cold dips in the room, for example, have some hot hors d'oeuvres in the oven, ready to be passed around. If you're serving a spicy curry, ensure there's a milder alternative for guests who don't care for it. Include some vegetarian and low-fat dishes, since food preferences vary widely. I usually have two desserts – one for the weight watchers, and another for those who want to indulge.

Be generous Having too little food can really put a dampener on people's party spirits. When working out your budget, allow for one or two spectacular dishes, such as a lavish prawn platter with dipping sauces, or a particularly luscious-looking chocolate dessert. That way, even if you're relying on lots of little sandwiches to make ends meet, you still create a big impression of festivity.

Do as much as you can the day before Most desserts can be made ahead of time; so can rice and pasta dishes and casseroles. Steer clear of fragile food that is not going to store well (souffles or meringue tarts) because such dishes are likely to get damaged if the fridge is full. Instead, store prepared foods in stackable plastic containers and decant them or heat them up on the day.

Cook in bulk Before you start preparing, compare the ingredients and instructions for the party dishes. Often you can double up by, say, chopping two lots of onions at once, thereby saving time and washing up.

The drink

It's rare to serve spirits at a party these days – beer, wine and champagne remain the most popular alcohol beverages to serve at parties. Here's how to plan your party purchases:

Work out quantities One 750 ml (24 fl oz) bottle of wine will serve six 125 ml (4 fl oz) glasses. Most guests will average between three to six drinks each (or about a drink an hour). If you are serving only wine, allow about half to a full bottle per person. Beer is more variable – allow about three cans or bottles per person.

Have a variety Offer two or three crowd-pleasing varieties, such as riesling and chardonnay for white, and a soft merlot for the red drinkers. If serving champagne for a toast, allow at least one glass per person.

Stock up on non-alcoholic beverages You'll need orange juice, bottled water (both sparkling and still), Coke or lemonade and perhaps a diet soft drink. Take the temperature and time of year into account, too – the warmer it is, the more liquid people will need.

Get ice Unless you have a fridge set aside for the purpose, plan on having someone collect at least two 10-kilogram bags of ice to fill the laundry tub.

Set up a bar away from heavy traffic areas, such as the kitchen. Use a fold-up card table to arrange glasses on and, ideally, have one person assigned to pouring and serving drinks instead of making it an open bar.

Such a little thing: finding time alone. Otherwise when is there time to remember, to sift, to weigh, to estimate, to total?

TILLIE OLSEN, POET

A last word

There's no getting away from it: life today is stressful. Surveys reveal that almost eight out of ten people suffer from stress, while seven out of ten have difficulty sleeping – one of the prime causes of stress. There's masses of information and a plethora of products out there to help you beat stress and take control of your life – books, tapes, CDs, DVDs, videos, relaxation products – so many, in fact, that it's stressful to consider them. Calming down is easier said than done. My favourite stress-buster has always been to laugh it off. Which is why I thought I'd share this piece that my cousin Liz sent me. I hope it puts your troubles back in perspective, too!

Try the following 'meditation' to reduce stress:

Close your eyes and picture yourself near a stream.

Birds are softly chirping in the crisp, cool mountain air.

Nothing can bother you here. No one knows this secret quiet place. You are in total seclusion from that crazy place called 'the real world'.

The soothing sound of a gentle waterfall fills the air with a cascade of serenity.

The water is sparkling and clear.

You can easily make out the face of the person whose head you are holding under the water.

Look. Why, it's the person who caused you all this stress in the first place.

What a pleasant surprise. You let them up . . . just for a quick breath as you breathe in, one, two, three . . . then, plop! . . . back under they go as you breathe out, one, two, three.

Allow yourself as many deep breaths as you want, dunking the person's head for as long as you like.

THERE NOW . . . FEELING BETTER?

Acknowledgements

Special thanks to:

My husband Doug, for giving me those long, fond, husbandly looks, for your calm and romantic nature, for meticulous laundry-folding, and for tireless bedtime reading aloud. You are my dream come true.

My sons Edward and Randall for being such wonderful, amazing, astonishing kids. You are courageous, funny, talented, affectionate, kind, and drop-dead gorgeous – better than I ever imagined.

My girlfriends Carolyn, Amanda, Vivienne, Eileen, Treg, Lesley, Lyn, Kerrie, Kezza, Suzanne, Nerida, Vickii, Shane, and all the BOGs – for the relief of having real conversations. You fortify my life.

My publisher Sue Hines, who merely has to walk into a room where an author is having a crisis of confidence and there is peace, vision and a positive direction.

The Dream Team at Allen & Unwin Andrea, Megan, Jennifer and April – and to Monty, Nick, Pauline and Dan – for your professionalism, diligence, good humour and punctuality. I feel so privileged to have had you all work on *Make Time*.

My agent Margaret Connolly, for being sensible, steely and darling, all at once.

*I am extraordinarily patient –
provided I get my own way in the end.*

MARGARET THATCHER

All the difficult things in the world must have once been easy; the great things must have once been small. Every thousand mile journey begins with a single step.

LAO TSE, CHINESE PHILOSOPHER